John

A Journey Back

Kevin J. Mallory and Nancy A Lane

iUniverse, Inc.
New York   Bloomington

iUniverse books may be ordered through booksellers or by contacting:

iUniverse
1663 Liberty Drive
Bloomington, IN 47403
www.iuniverse.com
1-800-Authors (1-800-288-4677)

ISBN: 978-1-4401-5546-8 (sc)
ISBN: 978-1-4401-5544-4 (hc)
ISBN: 978-1-4401-5545-1 (ebook)

Printed in the United States of America

iUniverse rev. date:08/26/09

Dedicated to

The Maine Children's Cancer Program

The Deering High School Class of 2010

The Make a Wish Foundation of Maine

Our Family, Friends ... and John

Contents

Acknowledgments

If the only prayer you said in your whole life is " thank you," that would suffice.

~ Meister Eckhart

On April 14, 2009, some months after John's journey had begun, I ran into one of my employees outside my office. She stopped me and asked quite pointedly, "Are you religious?"

I thought for a moment and responded with, "I'd have to say, not particularly. Why do you ask?"

"Well," she said, "I go to St Joseph's, and they are still offering prayers for John. Is John doing all right?"

With that, I thought about the first people for whom these acknowledgments are meant. This project began with the hope that John would fully recover, and, on graduation day 2010, I would be able to hand him as a gift this account of these troubled times. I also sought to include a look back at the memories that Nancy, my wife and John's mother, and I held so dear, so that, in ensuing years, our grandchildren (hopefully) would fully understand their father, his early years, the relationship he had with his parents, and his struggle. Developing the work made it clear to me that other people needed to hear and understand the challenges of childhood cancer as well. If this book contributes to at least one individual's education in this regard, I'll be pleased. For a parent facing a similar journey, my hope is that there are enough signposts in this book to help guide you and others through your struggle.

The past months have brought us in contact with many remarkable people. Simply saying thank you to these people seems inadequate.

Inevitably, we will forget someone. Please know that you are all in our hearts. Our friends, family members, colleagues, and a remarkable group of professionals who fashioned John's health care rose to new heights as, at times, they experienced the same pain we felt. The prayers and good wishes have been overwhelming and have carried the day when the darkness of early winter did its best to bring us down. Loving with no expectation of anything in return brought out a purpose in everyone close to John. We will always remember this notion and expect that, with the passing months and years, we can forever frame our lives in this manner.

Dr. Ann Rossi and the staff at the Maine Children's Cancer Program brought to us an expertise, compassion, and understanding when we were at our lowest. Without this unique group of people we would surely not have held together as well as we did through the process. During every visit, their smiles and observations made the experience real, yet, in a sense, normal. They held no agendas; their motivation was simply that they had the knowledge to beat the monster into submission, and that they would do just that.

The Barbara Bush Children's Wing at the Maine Medical Center produces magic in spite of the suffering of the young. To simply let children be children through a process that is so debilitating is their mission, a mission that they carry out with a dedication that impacts all who enter this special place of healing and spirit.

The Visiting Nurses Program was a godsend, and, without them, our lives would have been crazier than they were. Their weekly visit to draw blood kept John at home and was an integral part of managing fatigue after school when it was at its worst.

Our friends Joy O'Brien and Nancy Beaulieu took care of Nancy in a way only old friends know how to. Continue to be special. The beach will be calling soon.

Portland Public School Superintendent Jeanne Whynot-Vickers gave me unconditional freedom to stay involved with John and not have to worry about my work as Transportation Director. She epitomizes the difference between a real boss and those who only profess to know how to manage people. Keep the children in your heart as you move on. Well done!

Ken Kunin and his staff at Deering High School were professionally dedicated to making sure John got what he needed. This was such a tremendous boost. Their treatment of him as a normal high school kid made John's fight while at school that much easier and motivated him to do the best he could. To those who say teaching is just a job and not a career, they don't understand.

Dan and Tina Lucas helped us understand, guided us through decisions, and provided life-sustaining donuts. One day we'll sit on the beach again and laugh at Dan and John's stories while we watch the grandkids in the surf and age graciously.

"Aunti" Kaye Mallory had a silly thought about a stuffed bear. She gave the bear to John, and John smiled. The bear found a home. Sometimes it's that simple. Countless phone calls and servings of "aunti-pasta" raised our spirits and connected us with the family. When Uncle David falls under the evil spirits of the devil red wine, our gratitude for your care and feeding of him goes without saying.

Uncle David is not a dreamer; he's a realist. Thanks for grounding us. May your path be marked with the best wine and the time to drink it.

Jean Todd and Fraser Jones, we thank you deeply for always being there and sharing a meal with us. Friends never let friends go it along. We love you both for not allowing that to happen.

Judy Bichajian, you were John's guardian angel, and our personal relationship with you is such a good one. Thank you for helping me reexamine my faith in a new light. Your wisdom shone and, in some cases, carried the day for Nancy and I. The lake will soon thaw, the barbeque will crackle, and all will be right again with the world.

My staff is a group of individuals from all walks of life. It is no secret that they will never get rich from driving school busses. Like many people in education, they enjoy being around and caring for kids. With the challenges mounting up, this group of men and women were a blessing to be around. Your thoughtfulness, generosity, and kindness will be hard to repay.

Becky Bogdonavich is an amazing friend of Nancy's, and hell bent, it seems, on producing the most babies in the shortest period of time. It is inconceivable to me how, with your brood of small children along with your own personal suffering as you were diagnosed with breast cancer (at the same time John was diagnosed), that you found the time to cheer up Nancy with your humor and wit. A magnificent woman is what you truly are!

To Barbara Esposito—aka "Nana"—you are special. With a large family, including many grandchildren of your own, you continually sent flowers, phoned, and offered rides. And all of this to people you barely knew. This was a gift from someone we will never forget. You are one of the truly good people of the world.

Easing into middle age found me losing contact with many of my high school friends. Various reunions brought us all back together again. The forces gathered as the call went out. Thank you all for your concern and encouragement. Vicki, Mary Lou, Mary, Donna, and all of you who brightened our day through this ordeal. Let's grow old together, gang.

Rhonda Walker, Nancy's childhood soul mate, traveled far and never broke the bond.

The spirit of the dojo remained with the former members as their respect and caring for John never diminished with time. We bow to your concern and thoughtfulness.

Going beyond the language and offering compassion, Mrs. McGinty spoke to all that is good about teaching. I could have learned French with you I'm sure.

Tim Laman is contributing photographer for *National Geographic* magazine, and it is his photography that graces the front cover of this work. Tim, your kindness in contributing this piece, and the meaning it holds for John will always be appreciated.

As we traveled back and forth across the state of Maine many times, we formed a bond of friendship that among ourselves, when all is said and done, made the work that much easier. To my friends and colleagues at the Maine Association for Pupil Transportation (MAPT) please know that your thoughts and prayers helped us move forward continuously. To Lenny in particular, "I got you babe!"

We have never met Jan Howarth, editorial consultant to iUniverse online publishing, but it is due to her work that this manuscript is not just a set of ramblings. You could have just edited the work and took your check. You didn't. You coaxed the final product out of us in a way that said I want this to be a good piece. Your comments relieved our constant anxiety of sharing our thoughts. When you told me in your comments that "I think you have expressed events and emotions beautifully and elegantly," we were finally convinced that the time had come to move forward. Thank you for your expertise and guidance.

And, finally, the unexpected entry into our lives of the Make a Wish Foundation of Maine came at a time when John was just getting back on his feet. At first, John shunned receiving a wish from your organization. Although grateful, he felt embarrassed and offered, "I'm not dying; give it to someone who is." His words made us feel as if we had done our jobs as parents. With much prompting from us, he accepted your gift of a kayak, which will ensure that John has the opportunity to spend time in his favorite place, the ocean. There could have been no better gift from such a dedicated organization. Thank you.

Foreword

Each day in our lives brings to us moments that shift the present and influence the future with very little warning. For me as a high school principal, sometimes these have been moments of pride, like the unexpected phone call that informed me of a leadership gift to renovate the auditorium. Following this phone call, the hoped-for fund raising campaign became a reality, consuming hours with meetings, letter writing, and asking for support. Sometimes these moments have been a mix of amusement and bother, like the note with a link to a Facebook page that showed seventeen pictures in a group labeled "Second Block Bar-B-Que." Very considerately, one of the large group of students who cut class to grill burgers a block away from school labeled all the pictures with each student's name making our job that much the simpler. A few halfhearted protests later, all served a single detention, and we all now have an entertaining story to share of the clever and not-so-clever things our young men and women dream up.

Sometimes the moment comes in an e-mail that threatens dreams and serves to challenge our students, their families, and our teachers with a reality we prefer not to contemplate ... a reality we always assume happens to other people. Such was an e-mail that I received on Saturday, October 18, 2008—Homecoming Day—at 7:06 AM from Kevin Mallory, a friend, colleague, and the parent of a Deering student. Kevin was writing to inform me that his son John had been to see his doctor about a cough he could not shake. A chest X-ray, a CT scan, and surgery to remove enlarged lymph nodes for biopsy later, Kevin was letting me know that the surgeon and family doctor both suspected lymphoma, though the pathology report would not be complete until the following Wednesday. Kevin noted that John had not taken it well when he was first told, but "bounced back" as you will read in the compelling account that follows. Kevin asked that I prepare to tell John's teachers after the family knew for sure that John was diagnosed with cancer. He closed the e-mail noting that John was, "off to the dance tonight in his new duds."

I read the e-mail over several times during the course of the day on October 18, though I am not exactly sure why. I imagine I was preparing myself for speaking with John's teachers when the diagnosis was confirmed. Perhaps it was to help me come to terms with the knowledge, which I would need to keep private for a few more days as I went through a dance with new duds and a few school days with a secret cloud hanging over one of our students and his family. Whatever the reason, I went to the dance with a heavier weight on my mind than usual. But I was grateful that Kevin had shared his news with me so that I could help our school prepare to be of support if, and more likely when, the time arrived.

The following series of forty-six short chapters and an epilogue that you are about to read, and which I have also read over several times, touches me in much the same way the short e-mail from Kevin touched me on that Saturday of Homecoming. It is the direct and honest account of one family's journey in dealing with diagnosis, treatment, and whatever healing of the body and spirit was possible. It is not a series of lessons. It is not a set of suggestions to follow if your life finds you on the same path. It is John's story as seen through the mind and heart of a loving mother and father with the hope that perhaps the story will provide aid, comfort, and some light if cancer or some other life-altering and life-threatening event should visit.

Much has happened for John, his mother Nancy, and his father Kevin since this journey began. In this thoughtful and thought-provoking series of entries chronicling the events and placing them in the context of the life of their son, we are invited into the life of one family with honesty, humor, and humility. We are informed about details of cancer treatment and details of growing up with T-ball. We are asked to consider questions of medication and questions about how character is revealed. Throughout, we gain strength from family, from close friends, and from Tony's Donuts. This is not a how-to book instructing readers how to deal with challenge in family or life. Rather, it is a portrait of one young man, one mother, one father, one family, and one community that connects us all in our common humanity. We all will deal with the unexpected, unwanted, and undeserved as we live and learn. We all will be defined by our family, our experiences, our loves, and our friends. We all will gain and give comfort in many small ways that we pray will leave a legacy of caring, of concern, and of hope. This book is a gift given to future generations of the Lane and Mallory clans, their friends, and our community, who, as a result of the tale that unwinds in these pages, will all have a window into the lives of special people during a time of worry and distress.

It is a window we have looked through repeatedly since that e-mail was sent on the morning of the Homecoming Dance. As I spoke with John's teachers in the days following confirmation of the diagnosis, and as we continued to receive updates from Kevin and Nancy, we were united in our worry. Our job at school to support John was made easier by the timely and complete information we received from Nancy and Kevin. Our wish was that their job was made easier by the understanding, the flexibility, and the caring shown by John's teachers, Deering staff, and John's friends. As Kevin noted to me, one of the family's fondest memories will always be of welcoming John's French teacher of four years, Lynn McGinty, into their home. John had been in Ms. McGinty's class through French IV, and, as far as Kevin could tell, a bond had been made that was important to John and to Kevin and Nancy. To John's parents, Ms. McGinty's visit, her expression of concern, and her obvious warmth for their son meant that they were not alone. School would continue, John would connect to as much as his health and energy allowed, and his school and his teachers would keep teaching, keep caring, and keep hoping.

Our hope is that John someday will read these chapters, perhaps in no particular order, to a child, a grandchild, or just a friend who needs a story of caring and a sense of the connections that strengthen and bind lives together in times that challenge and try our souls.

Ken Kunin
Principal, Deering High School

Introduction

When he was a crawler he left your feet to journey to the sofa and bring you a ball. When he was a toddler he left your side to journey across the grass and bring you a leaf. When he was a pre-school child he left your yard to journey next door and bring you back a neighbor's doll. Now he will journey into school and bring you back a piece of his new world. His journeys are all outwards now, into that waiting world. But he feels the invisible and infinitely elastic threads that still guide him back to you. He returns to the base that is you, seeking rest and re-charging for each new leap into life.

~ Penelope Leach

When I first saw this quote, it helped me bring my rambling thoughts about John into a much clearer perspective. It helped me channel my focus through the process of dealing with John's illness as if it were a guidepost. It also brought parenting into a new light.

What we as adults see as rudimentary, a child sees as a journey of discovery. It is these individual journeys that start at birth and wind their way through countless phases, discoveries, and, yes, life-changing moments that fashion our children into who they eventually become.

As parents, we are surely drawn to this quote by the optimistic view that, no matter where the journey leads our sons and daughters, we as parents will remain the structure needed so badly by all human beings.

This brief narrative focuses on bringing the quote to life with a retrospective view of journeys past that define our son John as a person. His understanding of the world according to John, as with all teens, makes this story unique.

Through his journeys, he fashioned a soul. He would come to depend on this spirit time and time again as he battled to return from his toughest journey ever … the journey that began at the life-changing moment when he was told he had childhood cancer.

1

The Journey Begins

Until the day when God shall deign to reveal the future to man, all human wisdom is summed up in these two words,—"Wait and hope."

~ Alexandre Dumas

John's journey began on October 16, 2008, when he immerged from his doctor's examination room and, in a somewhat frantic gesture for a teenager, waved for his mom to come quickly. The physician's assistant met her at the door and quickly affirmed that John did, indeed, have bronchitis. She also stated that there were other issues of more immediate concern.

John's journey would involve many people, impact many people, and leave few people who know him unaffected. It would be a journey that would provoke a newfound sense of family, friendships, and caring. The focal point would not center on our shattered comfort zone of twenty-two years, but rather what had displaced it. We had no road map, no compass to steer by. This was a world of unknowns that would come at us with breakneck speed, posing a lifetime of questions in a very short time span that was not of our choosing.

The notion that "bad things happen to good people" was squarely there for us to confront. The reality of the moment was brought home forcefully; we felt as if we had been squarely punched in the stomach, and then punched again, and again. The times would test us more than any challenge we had faced thus far. The times would test our parenting skills, our faith, and our abilities to cope with something that, until

1

now, only happened to other people. For John, it would be a test of physical endurance and mental intrigue that would move him from one challenge to the next, willed on by his human spirit.

For all of us, the journey back had begun.

2

From a Physicians Point of View

Fifty percent of the doctors in this country graduated in the bottom half of their classes.

~ Al McGuire

Nancy called me at work to tell me what was happening. The conversation made no sense to me whatever. She rambled on and tried to explain to me what the doctor had told her.

"From a physician's point of view, this doesn't look good," was really all I heard.

"They said they want him to go for a CT scan, a chest X-ray, and have some blood work done. They want it done today."

Her monotone delivery was not Nancy. This was Nancy in distress mode. With an unspoken agreement between us never to call work unless it was something serious, I realized this was more than serious. With the phone buzzing and the radio blaring behind me, another interruption in my day was not a welcome moment, but I knew by the tone of her voice that I should listen carefully.

"What the hell are you talking about? I thought he just had a cough?" was all I could manage.

I wanted to be anywhere but where I was. I wanted to be beside them both. I take that back, I wanted to be beside Nancy at this moment. I knew John would handle this thing the way John handles everything. I could hear him now, "How long is this going to take?"

The rest of my day was a blur.

3

Nancy and Me and Baby Makes Three

A baby is God's opinion that the world should go on.

~ Carl Sandburg

John Lane Mallory was born May 23, 1991—our first and only child, adding to a family of two other boys from a previous marriage, both grown and out on their own. After five years of marriage, John was unexpected, but very much wanted when the news came. While we had never really talked about it a lot, I think deep down Nancy always wanted to experience being a mother.

So, here we were, two thirtysomethings, steady jobs, plenty of friends, and no inkling of what to expect except for my brief experience of earlier years with my first two children who had all-too-quickly left my life with their mother at a very early age. About to embark on an adventure that would change our lives forever, we mused over and discussed often just exactly what "Nancy and me and baby makes three" would mean to us. Well, it seemed to us we could handle it. I mean, how hard could it be? We'd seen people who had no business having babies do quite well, and whose children seemed no worse for wear. How much would it change our lifestyle? We'd worked in the business world for years and had taken everything they threw at us. We had watched as, all around us, friend after friend added to their families.

Final consensus: "What the hell, let's have a baby."

Soon after, the answers to our questions were apparent.

We were both nervous and excited to see who we were bringing into the world together. The nine months were fine on me and torture on

Nancy. Each day she swelled into something more and more resembling a beach ball. Getting in and out of bed was a test of endurance. Driving the car meant either laying her belly on the steering wheel or not using the foot pedals at all. No option there.

Nancy held a full-time job throughout, working as a sales representative for a major trucking company. Now understand one thing about this. She hated the job with a passion. Even dressed in your business suit and high-healed sneakers, it's hard to impress people who have as many teeth as they do fingers. She worked some of the most remote corners of the great State of Maine. She knew every wood manufacturer, and just what to pull out of the trunk of her car for their enjoyment and to garner a sale.

And now this added indignity. Waddling about the back country drumming up business was not what she wanted to be doing. But she did it—did it because we needed the added income that the package she was carrying certainly would require. And by Nancy's standards, there would be many needs.

You see, Nancy is a shopper. No, make that a world-class shopper. Shopping for her only child would be an experience that the faint of heart should avoid at all cost. She was methodical. Battle plan in hand, she would attack a store with the grit of George S. Patton and the tenacity of George Armstrong Custer. Leave no stone unturned, take no prisoners. Her child needed things. He would need lots of things. This was the thought process—nothing too good for him, and everything that other children had.

This was my wife—fat, smart, and untiring. Super Mom had made her first appearance.

What is it about childbirth anyway? You hear the old tales of women plowing the field, stopping to have a baby, and then finishing the north forty, and you think, *How the hell hard can this be?*

There are two things I remember not so fondly about childbirth. First and foremost, some advice: do not—and this bears repeating, *do not*—be tempted to hold hands with your darling wife during natural childbirth. You will not get back anything that resembles the hand you gave her.

Second, and equally important, try to remember that you are not a jerk, a jackass, or any of the other multitudes of names she will call you during this process. Delivering mothers don't mean what they say—really they don't. And it's not "your entire fault" either. What you are is the dutiful husband who is there to watch a miracle. Since you've chosen to be there while your wife is doing things that seem humanly impossible, and since she needs someplace to focus other than the ceiling tiles (remember Lamaze), who better than yourself. Let's face it, you can either suck it up or stay in the waiting room with all the other second- or third-time dads who value their hands and don't care all that much for obscene language from someone they have pledged their eternal love to.

Ours was a planned delivery. Think of that for a second. You make an appointment to go the hospital to have a baby. You know exactly when it's going to happen. No need to rush off in paint-splattered pants, or with hair leaning in every direction … you know exactly when the blessed event will take place. What a novel idea that is: induced labor. "Come on, honey, we're running late, we have to go have the baby now."

Anyone who has never gone this particular route before has got to be saying to each other, "that's the way to go." We have a plan, we have a timetable, perfect. Call the grandparents at two, baby at two-thirty, recovery until four, first feeding at seven, and, hell, I'll be home to watch the Giants by eight at the latest.

What was it someone once said about "the best laid plans of mice and men"?

The grand plan soon gave way to the shear panic of an unplanned cesarean section. Somehow this yet-to-be-born bundle of joy had turned himself in every direction except the one needed for a smooth delivery. The fact that he was hanging on to the umbilical cord added to the dilemma.

I had witnessed the predelivery technology of the birthing room before, so the machines hooked to Nancy that were monitoring her and the baby told me all I needed to know.

Heart beat racing, cervix not opening, baby in trouble … well, so much for natural childbirth. While Doogie Hauser and the other fresh-faced interns pondered, my mind raced as I watched Nancy on all fours doing whatever it was they asked of her.

Mustering up my best manners I asked, "Hello, um doctor, do you think this is good?"

In not too long a time, however, this pink resemblance of a child, covered with every imaginable kind of goop known to man, made his first appearance. When he'd been cleaned up a bit and handed to Nancy, we both beamed our satisfaction as the team went about doing their thing.

Then, finally, more panic. The delivery nurse, who up until that point I had barely noticed, made her presence known by proclaiming rather quietly, "Doctor, I don't like his color."

What, you didn't think I'd hear that or something? Off they whisked him, leaving us pondering another set of questions as the doctor proudly proclaimed, "Oh dear, you'll hardly see the scar at all."

4

Doctor D

Never go to a doctor whose office plants have died.

~ Erma Bombeck

When Dr. D says something, you listen. He's that kind of doctor. On top of that, when I first looked at him, I said to myself, *I hope this guy studied well, because I have a bald spot that's older than he is.*

Dr. D would always make it his practice not to condemn any of the bad habits you had picked up over a lifetime. He would, however, comment to the extent that he most assuredly made his point.

I smoke, and I drink. I'm not over the top about the first, but I am passionate about red wine. Our usual conversation during my annual physical proceeds something like this:

"So, you're still smoking?"

"Yes, Doctor"

"How much?"

"About a pack a day."

"Still drinking?"

"Yes, Doctor."

"How much do you drink?"

"Maybe a bottle or so of red wine a day."

"How much did you say?!"

"It keeps my cholesterol low."

"That may be, but so would one glass a day."

"I understand completely, Doctor."

"You also understand you're not getting any younger, and we've talked about this before. You need to start making better choices very soon."

"Thanks for pointing that out to me, Doctor. I'll see what I can do."

This was the kind of doctor I expected. Just let me make my own stupid decisions.

We would come to learn a lot more about doctors—many doctors, and very soon.

5

So, What Do We Tell John?

The truth is the only thing worth having, and, in a civilized life,
like ours, where so many risks are removed, facing it is almost the
only courageous thing left to do.

~ E. V. Lucas

To me, one of the most impersonal pieces of technology ever invented is the telephone. It eliminates the elements that eye contact and body language contribute to conversation. This is bad enough when you are speaking with people you know, but it is even more limiting when you are speaking to people you don't know. In my job, I answer the incessantly ringing phone for nine hours a day, so, when I arrive home into my sanctuary, a ringing phone becomes something for someone else to deal with. It could be at arm's length and I will ignore it faithfully.

I work for the Portland Public Schools as a Transportation Director. That is to say, I have responsibility for twenty-seven yellow school buses, thirty-two employees, and, most importantly, twenty-seven hundred children whom we transport from home to school and back again each day.

I had dark brown hair with a smattering of gray when I started the job. My hair is now completely white, with a distinctive bald spot in the rear. I've done this job for over thirteen years. To say I have seen everything kids who ride school buses can dish out is an understatement. It runs the gamut from the most ridiculous to the most heart rendering to the most stressful—and everything in between. There are days when I barely have time for a bathroom break, and days when it seems as if every life problem of everyone around me falls squarely in my lap. When the end of the day comes, the feeling can best be described as satisfaction with a just a bit of relief thrown in for good measure. Getting them there and home safely again is the hallmark of any good day in the school bus transportation business.

With the end of another day and with the popping of a bottle of red, I settled in and waited for Nancy and John, who somewhat unnervingly were not home yet from his medical tests.

When the phone rang, my immediate instinct was to just ignore it and let the machine take over. For some reason, unknown to me even now, I answered it. Doctor D identified himself and, without hesitation, started in on what he had to say. Then, as if he had broken rule number one of either his Hippocratic Oath, or, at the very least, company policy, he stopped and said, "I can tell you this because I assume your John's dad?"

"Um ... yes, Doctor, this is Kevin—your patient, and John's dad."

"We have some preliminary results from the CT scan and the X-rays, and it seems we are dealing with a lymphoma as I expected. Of course, we'll have to have a biopsy to know for sure, and I've gone ahead and set that up for next week. I was hoping Nancy and John would be home sooner so we could speak and I could answer any of her questions."

"Lymphoma?"

"Yes."

The rest of the conversation was irrelevant. I don't remember if I was rude, pushy, silent, or what. I remember he talked about it being treatable, good success rates, and good doctors.

"Treatable, success rates, doctors? Whoa, whoa, wait a second."

Cancer is the only thing I could focus on. John has cancer! My seventeen-year-old son has cancer! Are you crazy? My mind raced. He went in to be checked out for a cough. It's Thursday ... the weekend is almost here. He's going to the Homecoming dance for crying out loud! This isn't happening, this is some cruel doctor joke he's using to get me to quit smoking. Every stupid, unimaginable, and horrific scenario was playing out in my mind as I half listened. As he continued to talk, I heard the back door open. Nancy and John were soon in the room, and, without hesitation I asked Dr. D, "Nancy just came in. Would you repeat to her what you just told me doctor?"

John retreated to the television, and Nancy, as is her custom when talking on the phone, started wandering around the house. She said little, an occasional "yes" or "okay" followed by what seemed interminable minutes of silence. Nancy was absorbing the same news that had been given to me minutes earlier. The world that had crumpled around me was now coming down around her.

After hanging up the phone, she returned and sat across from me. She didn't cry, and she didn't speak. She just sat there, her already pale complexion now paler and making her appear old beyond her years. We both had the same information, and we were both slowly processing it.

"It's treatable, Nancy. They have good success rates"

"I know," she halfheartedly responded.

"He's going to be fine."

"I know."

"They don't even have a biopsy yet; it could be something else"

"He sounded pretty certain."

"So what do we tell John?"

"I don't know."

The moment had sunk in. The first tears fell as if on cue.

6

Why Do Babies Cry?

Babies are always more trouble than you thought—and more wonderful.

~ Charles Osgood

My dad would often remark to my mom with much candor, "Anytime I hang my pants on the bedpost, you got pregnant."

My brothers and sister grew up in what, by today's standards, was a large family of six children. Our mother was Italian Catholic, while Dad was of English-Scottish decent. Dad converted to Catholicism before the wedding, this being a part of the price to be allowed Mom's hand. We were raised, as my mother would say, "Not to be heathens, but good Catholic kids." With never enough money to go around, my parents did what I consider to be a remarkable job with what they had. Always, from their standpoint, the kids came first. There was never any question in regard to this.

Nancy was the younger of two daughters. She grew up fast, loosing her mother to breast cancer at age fourteen. She had no time to question why this had happened, only that it had, and it was time to move on. Her independent spirit was tested again and again as she fended for herself in a world that was not of her choosing, but one that her mettle would match stride for stride.

It was with this family backdrop that we arrived home with John. Anxiety and excitement both battled for our attention. Exhausted by the experience, Nancy rocked our newly arrived member of the family in his baby seat that warm day in May. The responsibility that lay before

15

us was sleeping, his eyes moving under his almost translucent eyelids. With just the slightest glint of a tear in her eyes, and with the deepest of sighs, Nancy exhaled and faintly remarked, "Now what do we do?"

With this one statement I thought about how woefully unprepared we were for this. Didn't you read the baby books, Nancy? What about all that advise from your friends? My mother, that's it, we'll call my mother. Then it dawned on me. I had experience with infants. I'd done the diaper thing, and the bottle thing. I knew how to stop them from fussing. This wasn't going to be that hard. We could handle it.

Somewhere, someone had given me the only piece of advice I ever remember about dealing with infants: They cry because they can't talk. They cry because they are essentially saying to you, "Hey, wake up, Mom and Dad. I'm either tired, hungry, or I need my diaper changed. I can't talk, so you figure it out." Knowing this upfront gives all new parents all the essentials they need to guide them through the process.

However, there is one other big reason that babies cry, and I believe it to be the most important. If you have narrowed the field with the above rotation, and the crying persists, I firmly believe that it's because the baby is simply bored. Babies want to be where the action is. To a baby, being held, entertained with silly faces, and cuddled is about the same as eating baked Alaska is to us. Babies crave attention. Come on, what else is there after you've stared at the mobile over the crib for two hours, and given up trying to understand how your hands sometimes disappear into the sleeves of your pajamas?

"Oh yeah, I'll play with Mom and Dad until I get tired; they won't mind!"

Don't ask me how, but infants also instinctively know when you are sitting down to a meal. They know exactly when a three-hour "who done it" movie is about to give up its secret. And sex—that's the topper. There isn't a baby alive who doesn't have a sixth sense that tells them when the time is just right for them to make their presence known. Look at the next infant who interrupts you when you're having sex. That little snicker you see is not gas.

7

John

The thing that impresses me the most about America is the way parents obey their children.

~ King Edward VIII

John is a lanky lad. Good looking, with more than a glint of the Irish devil in his eyes, John could charm anyone into believing he's the second coming of Christ if need be.

At seventeen, he boasted of his six-foot height as if it were a merit badge he had obtained. His five-foot-eleven-and-three-quarters height never, even soaking wet, held more than one hundred thirty pounds. Kids in my neighborhood growing up would have referred to him as a "bean pole."

Attending Deering High School in Portland with its rich diversity of multi-ethnic groups, John flourished as one of the many. The building itself is Old World architecture. Brick and stone, a clock tower, huge doors, and sweeping front lawns make it a formidable structure. Set in a middle-class neighborhood with just a touch of money, it speaks of alumni past as well as the challenge of today's youth. In his junior year, John, like many others before him, knew that he would soon leave this edifice for the unknowns of college and beyond.

His circle of friends included everyone from the star athletes to the stoners to the average high school kids who simply grew up in the neighborhood that he had known since grade school. Just a big bunch of lugs going about the business of being teenagers is their best description. They were going through the motions of high school as we had done before them, playing out the frequent dramas, and none of them had a clue that these would be the best years of their lives.

Now the girls, they were a different story. Somewhere in my collective high school memories there are a few girls who stand out as what the average guy would describe as "unreachable"; that is to say, "There is no way she is going to be caught dead with the likes of me." I can honestly say I have never seen John with anyone but this type of high school girl. They are all, quite simply, pretty. Not just cute, but pretty. Somewhere in the past forty odd years, I think God decided that high school boys had had enough, so he made all the high school girls pretty and said, "There now, have at it lads, let's see what you've got."

John was not an athlete to the extreme. He did what he wanted, on his own terms. John would participate in the sports he wanted to. Watching some sports rather than playing them spoke of his ability to fashion who he wanted to be. While I'm sure he always knew he could play the sports, there was always a little whisper in his ear reminding him that his one hundred thirty–pound frame knocking heads with guys who weighed two hundred twenty pounds was not all that good an idea. I'm sure that more than once the words "What are you, nuts?" rang in his ears.

Grades were easy for John. I should say grades were easy for John when John felt like doing the work and getting the work in on time. Still, he maintained an honor-roll average in all subjects despite driving his mom and dad absolutely crazy. High honors were not out of reach, but John would rather hang out then spend an extra hour studying. College … well, he'd think about that another day.

This was the child who, no matter what his parents threatened, cajoled, or otherwise did to make his life miserable at times, would saunter through his world with pretty much not a single care. He had his friends, his school, and his car privileges. He had a ready supply of spending cash (the parents who can't say no), and a nice girlfriend. In his world, he had a simple attitude that said to all who encountered him, "Isn't life grand?"

8

We Need To Talk, John

We swallow greedily any lie that flatters us,
but we sip only little by little at a truth we find bitter.

~ Denis Diderot

Amanda is a shy, soft-spoken girl with a little-girlish voice that I tease her incessantly about. She is also fast becoming John's soul mate. They spend every waking hour together that they can. So much so that I have kidded Nancy on occasion about her raising the daughter we never had. Today was like any other with her and John cuddled up watching television in the late afternoon.

"So what do we tell John?" I asked.

"I don't know," Nancy responded.

"The first thing you have to do is stop that crying. If he sees you like this, he's going to flip out and know something is really wrong."

"I know, I know, I'm stopping."

"We're only going to tell him what he needs to know—what we know: There is a possibility you have a lymphoma. They don't know everything yet, and, even if it is cancer, it's treatable."

"When do you want to do it?"

"We should do it now while Amanda is here. She can support him, and he'll probably hold it together. Let me do it."

So how do you tell your kid he may have cancer? How do you even prepare yourself for the hardest thing you'll do in your lifetime and the toughest thing he'll have listen to? Vacant are the sage words of wisdom fathers pass to their sons. All you have in this moment is the hope that you handle the event in a manner that is self-assuring and comforting, yet forceful enough so there is no misunderstanding. As we rose to move to the other room, we quietly came together in a hug that, for the moment, relieved the burden and reassured us both that John would handle this as he handles everything—in his own way, and on his own terms.

Cuddled on the couch before us they sat, absorbed in their latest television fantasy. We sat on the sofa opposite theirs, and I abruptly switched off the TV.

"Johnny."

"Dad."

"We need to talk, guy."

"About what?"

"About you and all the things you've been through today. So here it is. Doctor D suspects you may have a lymphoma."

There, I'd said it. I wanted to take back every word. This wasn't happening to us, and all I wanted was for this moment to go away. What in the hell had this normal, nice, average kid done to ever deserve this?

"Is that cancer?"

"Maybe, they have a lot more tests to do."

Amanda put her hand on John's shoulder as his head sank into his hands. I was totally unprepared for what I saw when he lifted it. I had not seen John cry since he was a baby, but here, today, the tears—huge dripping tears—poured from his eyes as if he had saved them all for just such an event.

Nancy quickly came to his rescue, and the three of them hugged and cried while I just looked on from the other couch, making no effort to join them. I couldn't—the guy thing held me back and kept telling me, he needs them, not me right now.

"I'm only seventeen."

The words came out of John so unexpectedly, I grasped for anything. *Just say the right words, find something, anything that will put those thoughts into the dark recesses of his mind for the moment.*

"That's right, and you're going to be eighteen, and nineteen, and twenty also," was the best I could do.

What did I expect from John anyway? I'd just told Mr. Carefree that life as he knew it, as we knew it, would never be the same. The terrible, terrible things that were going on in his mind at this moment were too much to comprehend. Cry John. Cry like you've never cried before if you want to.

There was nothing we could do or say at this moment except be with him as we had been through all the events preceding this horrific day. We, as parents, couldn't make things better this time as we had always done in the past. We couldn't make him safe from cancer. As I watched his tears subside, I thought to myself, *How mocking this is. Every day I am responsible for keeping twenty-seven hundred kids safe. Safe from bullies, safe from terrible drivers, and safe from all the crazy things kids do. Here in my living room, immersed in the reality of not being able to keep my own son safe from this affliction, I feel weak and useless.* It was an irony I would continue to revisit over and over again in the months to come.

9

The Little Man

Childhood is not from birth to a certain age and at a certain age the child is grown, and puts away childish things. Childhood is the kingdom where nobody dies. Nobody that matters, that is.

~ Edna St. Vincent Millay

Childhood, that is to say, the time when the infant stage can't fade away quickly enough, arrives upon parents all too fast. First walks, first words, the inevitable success of potty training … these are all milestones that rush by in a whirlwind and are celebrated in a manner akin to the pope having just bestowed sainthood on your mother. (I inquired, Mom. They said you had to be dead first.)

Mixed with these milestones is a learning curve that, for most people, is not as steep as one might think. Let's take ear infections for example. Where do they come from? Why do kids have so many? What's best, the pink medicine or the clear medicine? For average people to understand an ear infection, they need only know a few basic things. First and foremost, it apparently hurts. How do you know it hurts? The volume of the screaming will give you your first clue. How do you know what hurts? Well if they can't talk and they are furiously rubbing their ears, that should be the first clue. What medicine works the best? This is the key. The medicine that works the best is the one that finally stops the fussing after a couple of days. Yup, trial and error, even with ear infections.

You roll with the punches through early childhood. The first year is one revelation after another. Solid food is an adventure in and of itself. Now, you would think the simple act of getting a small spoonful of mashed something into the small mouth of a totally defensive child would be one of the easier things to accomplish. Ever see a child tell you that peas are not on his culinary list? A scrunch of the face and what looks to be an effort to blow bubbles with the peas ends in a scene reminiscent of the *Texas Chain Saw Massacre* (alien style—green blood!). So you try something else, saying to yourself, "Hey, I don't like strained peas all that much myself. I understand this."

Try as you might, you offer one food after another, but the bubbles still persist, the mess spreads further, and no amount of airplanes coming into the hangar or silly baby faces will end up helping you win the day. The salvation of the baby bottle awaits. Having now been totally beaten into submission by someone whose brain is like a sponge, but who can't utter the word "Dada," you mutter quietly to yourself, "Tomorrow is another day; you have to eat sooner or later."

10

The Bear

Don't be too timid and squeamish about your actions. All life is an experiment. The more experiments you make the better.

~ Ralph Waldo Emerson

Empty feelings of anger, denial, and uncertainly swirled within both Nancy and me. The surreal nature of the moment was eclipsing our ability to put things into perspective and think straight. Here it was Thursday night, and we'd know nothing until the next Wednesday when Dr. D had scheduled a consultation with the surgeon who would do the biopsy on John's lymph nodes. Left to ponder for six days if this was nothing or if John was facing an uphill battle for his life, we both found this totally unacceptable. With the urgency of the tests that day, and the tone of Dr. D, we knew it would be the latter and we weren't about to run on a doctor's, a hospital's, or anyone else's timetable. Not for one minute would we accept this as "downtime."

As quickly as the tears stopped, John appeared after an hour or so of talking with Amanda and declared, "Screw this. This is not going to interfere with my life. We're going to the dance Saturday night, lymph things or not."

Well, I guess he made that clear enough. I was so proud of him at that moment I simply said, "Cool, go to the dance."

Here he is, doing what I had hoped he would do. Putting on the game face and acting like someone who was treating this as nothing more than a common cold. Of course it wasn't a cold, and he knew that. He also knew that teenage things, at least for now, came first.

Nancy had already jumped into action mode soon after our conversation about waiting for news. As if by instinct, she knew exactly where to turn. Call someone who'd been through this. Find out what to do, what pitfalls to avoid, where to turn for advice, and what not to do.

Dan and Tina Lucas had been friends of ours for a long time. I met them through Nancy back when we had just started dating. They owned a real estate company and were parents as we well. Dan, a former professional hockey player, had recently experienced his own horrid bout with cancer—a cancer so severe it left him at times unable to talk, or even swallow. We had seen Dan battle for months to push this cancer into submission. His success was due in no small part to Tina and her efforts. She was a bear, never missing an opportunity to get Dan the right doctors or best treatment needed in his battle. From our standpoint, they had made all the right choices, and, as incredibly tough as it had been for their family, Dan stood as a testament to modern medicine, a loving wife, and a strong will. There could have been no better choice for us as we searched for someone to reach out to on this first day of our battle.

It was hard for Nancy to call Tina. She knew full well that, once again, Tina would have to come to grips with yet another person in her life having to experience another torturous climb from the bottom. As hard as it was, though, Nancy made the call and, without hesitancy, brought Tina up to speed.

You know the expression, "Friends don't let friends drive drunk." Well, there is another one I've discovered recently: "Friends don't let friends go it alone." Such was the case with Tina, and she made that abundantly clear with us. She and Dan were along for the ride, a ride they knew all too well, and a ride whose potholes along the way they had become all too familiar with.

Luck. Sometimes it's just plain dumb luck that carries the day. You get a break because you may be in the right place or you're there at the right time. Providence shines on you, and for no good or explainable reason, deals you a hand that couldn't have come at a more opportune time. For Nancy and I, the twist of fate occurred as Tina informed Nancy that she and Dan were acquaintances of the surgeon's wife who was scheduled to do the lymph node biopsy on John.

Without any hesitation, the bear took command of the situation. The fact that a mother, any mother, had to wait a week for this sort of news about her son was unacceptable to her as well. Tina offered to phone the surgeon's wife to see what could be done. I don't know this woman, but I know Tina, and I can only imagine the bear's conversation. At nine forty-five that evening, Dr. McGilvray called and told us to be ready the next morning. He didn't know what time, and explained there wouldn't be time for a consultation, but he'd fit us in.

The bear had roared.

11

Grandparents and Other Assorted Family Members

If you ever start feeling like you have the goofiest, craziest, most dysfunctional family in the world, all you have to do is go to a state fair. Because five minutes at the fair, you'll be going, "you know, we're alright. We are dang near royalty."

~ Jeff Foxworthy

I want to be a grandparent some day. Have you ever noticed the esteem that is bestowed upon grandparents? They are the great creators, the reason we all exist. Is it possible to fault grandparents? Of course we can, but does anyone ever have the audacity to get into a knock-down-drag-out with the creators? It's rare.

I want to be the kind of grandparent who can marvel at his grandkids one minute, and feel completely relieved as Mom and Dad take them home after a day of tickling them unmercifully and playing pull Granddad's finger.

Grandparents are a blessing, regardless of the often-ridiculous things they say and profess to know. I will not be that kind of grandparent. I will not discuss in mixed company my son's childhood bowel habits. Informing my son that his son should be a Democrat when he grows up or he'll rot in hell is not something I will do. Finally, I will not put the fear of God into someone who doesn't even understand how

Spider-Man soars from building to building. They have time for all that later.

Grandparents take anything thrown at them—divorce, illness, death, bad-mannered in-laws, you name it and they have a way of dealing with it all. In my family, if you aren't married and divorced at least once before age twenty-five, you risk becoming the black sheep. Six kids, thirteen marriages, thirteen grandkids, two great-grandchildren, and God knows how many ex-girlfriends, boyfriends, live-ins, almost marrieds, and assorted other folks have marched their way through my parents' life in the past years. You have to have a computer program just to keep the names straight. If we had a family crest, the motto on the bottom would probably read, "Don't get too friendly with them, they won't be around long." I'm not sure how that would translate to a few words in Latin, but in any other language it might simply read, "What were you thinking?"

I have a brother who actually had two girlfriends (at different times, of course) named Bambi. Outside of Disney World, I didn't even know this name existed, yet here in my family we not only had one, but two. We now refer to them as Bambi One and Bambi Two just to keep them straight. I thought one had a Corvette, but Nancy said that was someone else, so now I'm not sure who either one was.

Grandparents have a way of putting everything in a unique perspective. They tend to look at things that you'd think would have a great impact on them with nothing more than a "been there, done that" logic. Divorce? Seen it. New grandkid? Been there. To them, on the surface at least, everything seems like a big "ho-hum."

But—and this is the big but—don't ever, I mean ever, ever screw with the family. You screw with the family, you hurt one of the kids in any way, or put them on the spot by making them have to choose, and the logic immediately gets turned to, "Been there, done that, and now watch me do it with horns, missy."

That's the place I want to be when I'm a grandfather. The great creator, wise beyond my years, with my kingdom intact, my family prospering, and just enough in-laws so I never have to ask, "What the hell was her name anyway?"

12

Hospitals

We cannot be properly ill in a hospital, nor die in one decently; we can do so only among those who love and value us.

~ Thomas Szasz

It is rare that the word *hate* slips into my vocabulary. But it best describes my feelings toward hospitals. Hospitals are where people go to die. Hospitals smell. Hospitals offer degradation after degradation. Hospitals are slow and plodding, and run only on their own detached time.

Apprehension overwhelmed me as I left work and headed to the Maine Medical Center. John and Nancy would be waiting at the day surgery unit. They were still waiting for what should have been a two o'clock procedure when I arrived after four and met my very testy wife, equally bored son, and his visually nervous girlfriend. John was supposedly next on the hit parade, as the doctor was just finishing up with his last patient.

Time stood still as the four of us killed time in our own little worlds. People came and went. The waiting room fast emptied as fewer and fewer souls remained. Had they forgotten us or something? Was this going to be my typical hospital experience again? Finally, after what seemed an eternity, our turn came as two nurses appeared to explain the "pre-op" procedures. Off we went to this next phase—another unknown for us, yet a simple normalcy in the everyday working world of a hospital.

The process was now picking up speed. With any number of nurses entering and exiting, explaining things, attaching intravenous contraptions, and passing us forms to signs, the room was a buzz of activity with each participant focused on his or her particular job. Now this was more like it.

Soon the anesthesiologist arrived to ask his set of questions and explain what was going to happen. The nurses had sedated John to relax him for the surgery, and he explained to us that John might act a bit goofy, laugh a bit, and carry on in silly manner. John's ears perked up.

He soon reacted with all the aforementioned mannerisms and giggled incessantly each time he spoke.

When it came time to wheel John to the operating room, the nurse announced almost casually, "Okay, time for kisses and hugs. John has an appointment now."

First myself, then Nancy, and finally Amanda each said our awkward good-byes as if John were simply going off to college rather than for surgery. As they wheeled him off, our eyes met. With a silly little grin, and a "Later, dude" John slapped me a high five, and he was gone.

13

Daycare

If you bungle raising your children, I don't think whatever else you do well matters very much.

~ *Jacqueline Kennedy Onassis*

If there is one aspect of raising children that far and away tests the will of young parents, the daycare situation is it. For most two-income families such as ours, there are few choices. Without a friend or a family member to watch your children, you cast them into the sea of childcare providers and are left quivering at the thought that you have to give up your child once a day to a person who has ten or twelve other mouths to feed and bottoms to diaper, and hopefully has enough energy to spread a caring attitude toward each task.

Infant daycare is the first of the age-appropriate daycares in the evil empire of the daycare world. We researched, asked friends, did site visits, interviewed, and ultimately used our gut feelings to guide us. Did we like the director? Was the facility clean enough? What about the staff? Why are so many kids crying here anyway? All you can do is the best you can. Instincts rise above all else. Angst follows you the entire time. Leaving your baby with a complete stranger is not a natural act for a new mother. It's scary at first, and always leaves you questioning if you made the right choice.

Trust me, this too shall pass.

There are things you must understand about most daycares. First of all, people run them because they generally like kids, and like being around them. People run daycares for income opportunities, and, in a lot of cases, they run them to just be able to be around their own children. This is the sort of daycare you need to latch onto, especially with infants. Forget about the "factory" daycares, you'll have plenty of time for those later. Daycares who accept very few children are the best. Providers are less likely to put your child on a waiting list when the child needs something.

Money? Forget about it. Don't bargain, pay them what they ask. This is your child we're talking about here—you're not trying to buy a used Volkswagen.

Thinking back on daycares now, I'd like to think we did okay. A rocky start culminated with John making relationships with lifelong friends, becoming more independent, and, in some sense, becoming a more rounded individual. You'll cry the first few times you leave your child, and revel in the tales of providers later as they tell you about the day they had. Someone's kid will eventually punch yours, yours will have a meltdown over nap time, and sooner or later he'll get a "time out." And you know what? He won't be any worse for the wear of it. Oh, and stop beating yourself up because we don't live in 1950 with Ozzie and Harriet. David and Little Ricky would have faced daycare if Harriet had been forced to work!

14

A Second Opinion

Opinions are the cheapest commodities in the world.

~ Author Unknown

In what once had been a packed waiting room outside recovery, now only a few souls lingered about. Nancy sat alone after I returned from taking Amanda home. As I sat next to her, we both stared at the screen that listed the patients' progress from prep to surgery to recovery. The screen was the center of everyone's attention; we felt as if we were waiting for an airplane arrival at a busy airport: "Now arriving in Recovery Room C we have Mr. Jones fresh from his skin biopsy. Please proceed to the desk for further instructions."

"It says he's in recovery now, Nancy. Can we go see him now?"

"No, we have to wait for the doctor to come out and speak to us."

More waiting and more silence. We were both deeply lost in thought as Dr. McGilvray came from nowhere and leaned in saying simply, "Hello." Nancy jumped at his unexpected presence as if shot out of a cannon. Embarrassed by her response, she soon hung on his every utterance. "John is fine. There were no issues with the procedure. There's a room over here where we can talk."

As we settled into the small room meant for just this occasion, I introduced myself as John's dad and thanked the doctor for helping us. He looked tired, but his eyes held an intensity that spoke to his focus on the moment. The small talk was minimal, with all of us simply wanting to push on with it.

"It appears we are dealing with a lymphoma. Of course, they'll still have to send the specimen off to the lab. We should probably have some results by Wednesday. John has an appointment with me on Wednesday, and we'll talk more."

Dr. McGilvray possessed a simple and straightforward manner. This was, in all likelihood, the same conversation he'd had hundreds of times with other people waiting for an answer they didn't want to get. Nancy flinched as I touched her shoulder just enough to let me know she knew I was there. Without saying a word, she pulled away as if to say, "Not now, I need to listen."

The doctor told us where the cancer was located. He reiterated what Dr. D had said about it being treatable. He spoke about the just completed procedure of removing some of John's abnormally large lymph nodes for biopsy. An explanation soon followed about the relevancy of this. He remarked about the rate of success in patients in John's age group. His manner spoke of the confidence in a procedure that his profession had mastered for just such diseases, and for people just like John. There was no sugar coating, no attempt to downplay anything, just an explanation that he had repeated many times before.

Dr. McGilvray is a surgeon. One the best surgeons, he had done this procedure many times before. His opinions had been confirmed with pathologists an equal number of times. He knew he was rarely wrong and spoke in a manner that said so. But still, he was a surgeon and not a pathologist.

And, just like that, he was gone. As we sat in the small room pondering the information we had just received, we both seemed almost relived to finally know what were dealing with, yet we both secretly held out hope that he was wrong. No amount of explanation or logic could trump our still-glimmering hopes. We'd outlast them all until the final rendering.

We had one more chance to make this whole thing go away. We could still cling to the chance that we'd awake from this horrible dream and return to Saturday night dances, laundry piling up, and all the other inane moments of family existence that seemed so normal, yet, on this night in October seemed so very far away.

15

Of T-Ball and Worms

We all believe that our children are the most beautiful children in the world. But the thing is, what no one really talks about is the fact that we all really believe it.

~ Heather Armstrong

My father never came to my football or baseball games. With six mouths to feed and no time for anything but work, it was no wonder. It still hurt though. I wanted him there. I wanted him to see me at my best. I held up well in these sports, and, in some areas, even shone. I know he would have been proud to see me hitting a homerun or catching a touchdown pass.

This would not happen to my son. It was out of the realm of possibilities. I'd take every opportunity to make sure he got involved, and that I would be there to witness every historic moment of his athletic prowess. And I'd make sure he started early enough so that he would get all the proper coaching he needed to one day land him a full-time job with the Boston Red Sox.

Have you ever witnessed a T-ball game? Well, to call it a game is certainly a reach. I don't even think they keep score. To play T-ball in Maine, you must be ready to play in the semi-frigid conditions that are present on many game nights. Parents, grandparents, and neighbors are still bundled with parkas while half-frozen children stand in the outfield proudly displaying their T-shirts emblazoned with the name of the local hardware store. More than once I'd proclaim to Nancy before the end of some serious T-ball, "I'm frozen, I'm out of here." Super Mom would never dare.

I don't think that John ever enjoyed T-ball that much. On the off chance that he did hit the ball off the tee and it made it past the pitcher, he'd just turn around, look at us, and smile while the entire opposition ran after the ball resulting in what best can described as a "free for all." In running the bases, he did not fare much better, as more than once John sprinted from home to third base with a frantic coach chasing him. It amazed me that somehow he was always safe at first in the end.

In the field, John would spend lonely hours either watching airplanes from the nearby airport or searching for worms, which always seemed to find their way home with him in his pants pockets. When a ball was hit in his direction, John would look around with a quizzical look on his face, as if to say, "What the heck is everyone yelling about?"—until he noticed that the entire team was charging in his direction. "Oh yeah, the baseball!"

John participated in baseball reluctantly for two more seasons and eventually declared while freezing one day, "This is the most boring sport ever."

Well, so much for baseball, and so much, it seems, for the Boston Red Sox.

16

Bedside Manners

I am still determined to be cheerful and happy, in whatever situation I may be; for I have also learned from experience that the greater part of our happiness or misery depends upon our dispositions, and not upon our circumstances.

~ Martha Washington

John was still groggy from the anesthesia. I looked down on him and didn't see a teenager—he was John the little boy again. He appeared pained and spoke in hushed tones, his mother by his side tending to his helplessness. How many more times would a scene such as this rewind in the coming months? How many more moments such as this would we have to endure as modern medicine took over and shunted us to the sidelines?

As if knowing by the look on our faces, John broke the silence and reminded us that he was still John. Amazed that it was all over, he was again the seventeen-year-old … again the wise-cracking, irreverent, unpretentious John. "They never even asked me to count to ten, Dad!"

"This isn't television, John."

"Well, it stinks. I wanted to count to ten."

"Well, maybe next time."

This was the part of being in a hospital I had come to loathe. I'd been here before. A mother with a breast cancer scare, a brother with a brain aneurism that nearly killed him, and three childbirths had made this an all-too-familiar place. And I can't forget the father-in-law who fell off a ladder—Nancy had her own memories of this place.

The room was awash in activity. Nurses and doctors flew about oblivious to the small curtained rooms that each held a story. If such a thing as a human factory were possible, I suppose this was it. The old, the young, and everyone in between were here for whatever surgery the doctors had recommended.

John knew nothing about what the doctor had told us earlier. There wasn't any good reason to rehash with him what he knew to be a possibility. He was exhausted from being here for so long and simply wanted to go home. More vital signs, more checking, and more questions started to make him cranky. Who could blame him? It was Friday night and here he sat. He wanted to be with his friends and Amanda. This was an unwarranted break in his teenage routine, and he hated it. "When can we leave, Mom?"

"When they tell us you can, John."

"I feel fine."

"John, you just had an operation."

"So?"

"So just relax and stop playing with the bed, John." I offered, wanting to change the subject.

"It's cool; we should get one of these."

"Watch some television, John."

"Television sucks here. They don't have all the channels."

"I'm sure they have something you can watch."

He soon lost interest with the television and went back to trying to convince anyone who would listen that his Friday night was melting away. With all the bluntness of John being John and loud enough so that anyone could hear he proclaimed, "This sucks, Dad."

"Yes, yes, it truly does suck, John."

17

Bobble Heads

Sports do not build character. They reveal it.

~ Heywood Broun

Football is an oasis for me. For one day a week in the fall, I can remove myself from all the necessary wants and worries and plunk my expanding waist in front of my oversized television to revel in the painstaking adventures of The New York Football Giants.

When television was in its infancy, and prior to the games of the upstart American Football League being broadcast nationally, the Giants were the only team shown on television in Maine. Each Sunday, I'd gather with my dad or brothers to watch the black-and-white sameness of a team that never seemed to make good on its promise of "wait till next year." I learned the game of football watching the likes of Y.A. Tittle, Rosey Grier, Spider Lockhart, and a cast of characters who, throughout the early '60s, never failed to disappoint.

John got the bug early. Nancy was pregnant with John when, in 1991, lightning struck the Lawrence Taylor Giants a second time. With the Giants winning the second of two Super Bowls with a last-second field goal, Giant blood flowed freely through John that day.

Organized football was never available to us when we were young. You had to wait impatiently until the seventh grade. Then you could finally don the armor and challenge yourself to play the game you thought you knew so much about. Before that it was simply choose up sides and point out what bush was out of bounds. As darkness swept over us, we'd play until someone declared, "Last touchdown wins."

Bruised and sometimes bloodied, we'd return over and over without pads for protection until the first snows of winter tried in vain to chase us inside. This was football in the purest sense.

While winter stopped us from sure-handed catches, it did not force us to put the football away. Unwilling to use snow as an excuse to give up what had kept us busy all during the fall, we simply created another frolic to test our youth. "Kill the guy with the ball" was a simple game. Well, to call it a game is unfair. This event was pure survival. Simply, the kid who came with the football tried to keep it for as long as possible. He was the guy with the ball, and killing him was the goal. Bad terminology, but nonetheless fairly accurate when six or seven guys finally caught the poor guy and tried wrenching the ball away. Having lost sight of the sky while being crushed on the bottom of the pile, the guy with the ball would eventually give it up. He had been officially killed. On it went until we were soaked and frozen and, one by one, had dropped out. Winning didn't take much; you simply had to be the last person holding the ball. As we trooped off to the warm confines of our homes, it also became apparent that the usual winner was the person with the most layers of clothing. The game did have one caveat. Freshly fallen snow—not ice, and certainly not slush—was the best condition for this game. Although, from time to time, we attempted to play in ice and slush.

John was lucky—for him, organized football began in elementary school. By the time he was in the fifth grade, local youth leagues had sprung up over the years to cultivate a new crop of Portland gladiators to feed the middle schools, who in turn fed the high schools. The weeding out of kids thrown to the lions this young would soon occur. Bodies on the scrapheap of football rejects soon piled up, even at this tender age. Whether because of the lack of measurable skills or a body simply not meant to play football, many kids reasonably deduced early that a baseball glove was in their future.

When I first saw the kids decked out in practice gear, I laughed. Here was this group of midgets wearing football pads, ideally made for their size. The helmet was a different matter. The vast majority of these kids had one thing in common. They were skinny. Oh, don't get me wrong, there were some so overweight they waddled. But it was the skinny kids with these football helmets that made them appear for all the world like the bobble head figures of their favorite sports heroes. They just seemed to have enormous, wobbly heads.

The few kids who had any skill—or happened to be a coach's son—were soon the kids who would handle the ball. The lines were a collection of fat kids as well as marginally overweight kids. Defensive back or linebacker was the fate for the remainder. The best of the bunch also got to play both ways. John settled into his role as wide receiver with an enthusiasm and a gusto we had never seen in his baseball playing days.

He loved football. He loved being around the guys, and being part of the team. His teams were successful also. As he played on undefeated teams as a sixth grader and again his eighth grade year, we were there for every game, every moment. As much as he liked his football, his body told him otherwise. Knocked unconscious and hauled off to the hospital as a sixth grader, and then missing a lot of time due to injuries in his eighth-grade year, John slowly came to the realization that his one hundred odd pounds would not carry him to a high school career unless he ran like hell and no one ever caught him. But John was of average speed, and his football career came to an inglorious end with John just being John and offering, "Gee, Dad, it's only a game."

Yes, John, you're right … it is only a game.

18

Homecoming

The young know how truly difficult and dreadful youth can be.
Their youth is wasted on everyone else, that's the horror. The young
have no authority, no respect.

~ Anne Rice

John and Amanda had anticipated the homecoming dance for days. It was an opportunity to step out of the norm for both of them, to get dressed up, to be with their friends, and, heaven forbid, if not act like adults, at least resemble them for one night.

Amanda had shopped in Boston with her stepfather for the perfect dress, hoping to find something mature, and, in her own words, "Not slutty like all the other girls wear." She did not disappoint in the least. The strapless, black-and-white number she purchased seemed made just for her. It was made to impress, and indeed did just that.

Teenage boys have this peculiar habit of knowing how to make themselves look good, but never wanting to do so. John's typical attire consisted of T-shirts, baggy pants, sneakers, and the occasional hat that usually had to be turned sideways. We'd just shake our heads and continue time after to time to insist he, "Put a belt on." The problem was, he had a belt on. He was just so damn skinny that the end result was always that his pants sat six inches below his waist.

Tonight would be different. Nancy had spent the better part of a week trying to find a suit for John. Through all the tragic turmoil of this first week, she had made a point of making sure that, if John wasn't feeling well, she would surely make sure he was the best dressed boy not feeling well. Her hunting bore fruit when she succeeded in finding John a dark Calvin Klein vest and trousers for the special night. She refrained from buying the jacket thinking the vest would give him the look John was aiming for—not too dressy, but still able to compete with Amanda, and, more importantly, look good for her. The new clothes called for a trial run. As he came out of the bathroom dressed in his new duds, I was amazed at the transformation. It was rare to see John like this, and he looked very, very nice. Of course, my moment was short lived when John announced, "I look like a waiter." Nancy, alias Super Mom, never flinched. While I was ready to drive home the point that maybe saying thank you to his mother would have been a better opening, she merely offered, "Do you want the jacket?"

Saturday night came all too soon for Nancy and me. We knew it was the right thing to do, the normal thing, to allow John to head off to this dance. We just couldn't deal with the conflicts of his recent surgery. He had just been cut into yesterday. Is this good for him? Shouldn't he just rest? What if the guys get horsing around and he has issues with the wound? As much as we were happy to see this night come off for both of them, our apprehension was at times overwhelming.

With the jacket, the suit looked like any business suit you'd see on any professional anywhere. No, it looked better. This handsome kid made it look like a tailored suit. The vest was snug at his lean stomach; the pants the perfect length. He even appeared to have shoulders in this suit. I tied his tie for him and folded a handkerchief for his breast pocket, much the way fathers have done for sons for decades. He was Mr. GQ tonight. He was not just one of the boys in the hood tonight. He was the one with style. Oh yeah!

As Nancy and I ushered him off to pick up Amanda and return for pictures, the silence became noticeable to both of us. We both were thinking the same thing: He has cancer. How can somebody so sick look this good? How do we push those thoughts into the recesses of his mind and continue to act unfazed? What's he really thinking about? Does he actually comprehend what's going to happen to him in the coming weeks? Maybe he does know. Maybe he knows more than we think. Is he thinking tonight might be his swan song? Is tonight the night a teen rationale takes over and he says to himself, "Screw it, it is what it is, and, if it has to happen, this is how I'm going to be remembered."

When John and Amanda appeared together, it was every parent's special moment. Cast in the light of adult clothing, these kids exuded a charm and grace that belied the fact they were only seventeen. They glowed, while still maintaining the youthful giggles and gushes that made them who they were. This was their night to share and revel in.

After the pictures, we gave them all the perfunctory advice we could about driving, drinking, and what time to be home. Then we led them to the door. We were happy for them, happy they could have this one special, normal night before the turmoil that we knew would encompass both of them.

Nancy cried as they drove off.

19

Jelly Sandwiches

*Part of the secret of success in life is to eat what you like
and let the food fight it out inside.*

~ Mark Twain

Everyone tells the parents of young children that the eating habits those
kids establish when they are young will help provide solid footing for
the way they approach food as an adult. Feed them broccoli as a child,
and chances are they will eat it as an adult.

As the infant years rolled to toddler years and beyond, it was
apparent that John had made up his mind to be a somewhat finicky
eater. He'd munch the occasional healthy carrot or apple, but his food
interests were not what one would call "satisfyingly healthy."

John survived almost entirely on jelly sandwiches for lunch and
chicken nuggets for dinner for three years. Not just any jelly sandwiches
or chicken nuggets. His palate would accept formats of only seedless
raspberry jelly on white bread and Weaver chicken nuggets. Place a jam
or marmalade sandwich in front of him, and it would remain on his
plate with one bite taken. Change the brand of nuggets, and you'd get
a blank stare.

We both felt guilty. Would our friends find out and turn us in as
bad parents? Would the pediatrician shame us on each visit? Hey, we
tried. We experimented, and occasionally had some success.

John's scores always landed in the appropriate size and growth
percentiles, and we always told his pediatrician of his diet. Her
comment, "Well, he's growing just fine."

Hamburgers, hot dogs, and French fries soon followed, all smothered with horrendous amounts of ketchup. He was branching out—an apple here, and a pear there. Did I say pear? Only if it was rock hard and contained no juice, of course. Macaroni with red sauce, at first without the sauce, soon became a staple. John's eating habits drove both of us crazy at times. He would like one food today, and not like the same food tomorrow. We soon took to asking him what he wanted for dinner, but when the answer came back nuggets time and again, we accepted our fate. Mr. Consistent had spoken. Nuggets, oh nuggets … the dinner of champions.

20

Odds

Life is a gamble, at terrible odds—if it was a bet you wouldn't take it.

~ Tom Stoppard

Tuesday, October 21, 2008, was just another day in the waiting process. I went off to work as usual, and Nancy stayed home with John.

People are well intentioned and often speak from the heart when they inquire or offer to help. They'll submit over and over such encouragement as, "Try to stay busy," "Keep your chin up," and "We know he's going to be fine." People are concerned, and, even if you've explained your situation until your head hurts, you will need to explain it again. They deserve it. All the while, your heart breaks each time you relive it. While you try to stay upbeat when they ask how John is doing, a little piece of you dies each time. I don't think I've been all that good at it. I think people have seen through my answers.

Dr. Anne Rossi is cast from the mold of today's doctor. She has never once fallen back on any supposed comfort lines, but has always made us feel comfortable. As a doctor, she is analytical, soft spoken, but straight forward. I don't know where she went to school; I don't care. I didn't care what her qualifications were. She works for the Maine Children's Cancer Program. She had seen it all. She is a specialist who has managed childhood cancer in children of all ages. She was our doctor. More precisely, she is John's oncologist.

Our first exposure to Dr Rossi was when she called Nancy and explained that, although the pathology had not come back yet (our third opinion), she was quite sure that John had a lymphoma, and that he was in stage four.

"Stage four, what the hell is stage four?" But I knew all too well what it meant when Nancy called me with the latest bad news.

Quite simply, it meant that John's cancer had moved from his lymph nodes to other parts of his body. This was a whole new ballgame. It was as if this insidious trail of events was heaping more and more unfathomable things onto us to contemplate. Stage four? He had a cough. How in the hell did we get to this? You're telling me that this has spread? You're telling us that his major organs have now come into play? Now what?

On Thursday, October 23, 2008, we met with Dr Rossi for the first time. She was not in the least what I expected. She was striking. She was tall, but not overly so. She dressed most fashionably, and every hair was in place. But, most importantly, she offered a smile that brought a measure of comfort to us as we listened intently to her thoughts.

She talked about the disease and what we could expect. She explained John's treatment program, a regiment designed exclusively for him. She allowed us to ask any question and listened attentively when we asked them all.

John would have the standard treatment for childhood Hodgkin's lymphoma. There was no need to go to Boston or anywhere else. John would receive the same cocktail of drugs researched and developed precisely for this type of cancer. John would be a pediatric patient of the Maine Children's Cancer Program, and they would exclusively manage his care. Everything done from this point on would be in the hands of these people on whose office walls hung the pictures of thousands of bald, smiling children.

I didn't want to ask the question, but it lingered on my lips for what seemed an eternity. How would John react if she gave us anything but encouraging news? How would Nancy rise to the latest in a set of challenges that she had, until now, beaten back with a veracity that only a mother protecting a child could fathom.

"Doctor ... um ... I know it's too early to talk about prognosis of any kind. With this kind of treatment, can we talk about success rates ... survival rates?" For better or worse, the cat was out of the bag.

"Well, it's different for each age group, but we've had good success with this treatment, and, if it doesn't work as well as we think, we can alter things. But 70 to 85 percent is the result we usually achieve."

My mind raced. I thought about football, horse racing, poker—anything that odds were offered against—and tried to tie them together in a manner I understood. For some strange reason, I thought about placing four quarters on a table, and then taking one away. These were good odds, encouraging odds. These were odds that, if there had to be odds, I could accept and deal with.

John never moved. He looked stoically ahead as she spoke. I watched, and I thought I knew surely what he was thinking. He was soaking it all in as he sat on the edge of the examination table. He understood her words and realized the meaning of the numbers she had offered. I hoped with all my heart he'd see the odds as something encouraging for the first time.

So we had a plan, we knew what to expect, and we had met the team that would guide us on the journey that had started barely a week earlier. The best doctors, the best medicine, and the best facilities—all the knowledge and expertise and resources would combine to fight alongside us to beat this affliction. We felt relieved, while at the same time a bit overwhelmed by a system that, until now, we had never heard about. The program's manual, aptly entitled *A Journey of Hope,* would now become part of our personal journey. There was no way that together we wouldn't be successful. No way!

21

Mans Inability to Otherwise Act Normal

Men live in a fantasy world. I know this because I am one, and I actually receive my mail there.

~ Scott Adams

If the male teenage hormones (probably the female hormones as well) could speak to a teenager, they would probably say something like this: "Okay, guy, you got these things called hormones, right? That's me. We can be a major pain in the ass what with your voice changing, peach fuzz growing, and mood swings, but you know something? We can also be really, really fun! What, you want proof you say? Okay then, take that fine-looking young lady over there. Yes, the one with the short blond hair. Now I ask you, before I came along, what did you think? Right, not much you say. Now look at yourself. Are you sweating? That's me, buddy. I can do that you know. I can make you do that when you see a pretty girl. Oh yeah, I got other things I can make you do also. Now, clear your throat and go talk to her."

Hormones—they are all that is needed to release the hounds.

Don't get me wrong, having been married three times, and having had more relationships that I care to remember, my hormones have led me through more twists and turns than any man should have had to endure. Truth be told, I enjoy being around women. In some sense, I enjoy being around women more than I enjoy being around men. The

Mallory gene is likely responsible for this hormonal imbalance. Make that the *evil* Mallory gene. In possessing this gene, John would soon fall victim to what I refer to as "man's inability to act otherwise normal in the presence of a captivating female."

Men don't plan it this way. Middle-aged men normally can talk candidly about most any subject put before them. Normally guys could care less about a stain on their T-shirt. We stand up straight and belch with the best of them when conversing with other men, with or without wives or girlfriends present. Now, put Halle Berry in the midst of a bunch of paunchy middle-aged men and watch the meltdown. The brave will stay. Others will simply skulk away. Mouths become dry and intelligent talk fades from the scene. Symptoms include but are not limited to: stomachs sucked in, wandering eyes, and fantasies running rampant. See what I mean? "Man's inability to act otherwise normal" has now taken center stage.

Now, if middle-aged men after years of being conditioned, and whose hormones, let's say, don't have the ability to "kick it up another notch" respond this way, what chance does a teenager have against the forces of nature? Answer: zip, zero, nada!

With the Mallory gene and his already raging male hormones, John didn't stand a snowball's chance in hell of surviving the first eye contact cast his way. He was destined to act this way over and over again much as has forefathers had done before him.

John did not disappoint in this regard, but he did surprise us—at least me. Through an assortment of teenage adventures, John held fast to his best friend. This was a best friend who was never at odds with his hormones and someone who never made John succumb to "man's inability to otherwise act normal." Her name was Ashley.

This petite blonde pixie was every inch the tomboy, and at the same time possessed more than enough charm and feminine attributes so that there was no mistaking she was all girl. We took to calling her the "queen bee" because of her ability to gather others about her in a manner that most kids didn't possess.

John and Ashley met in the very early years of elementary school at a daycare run by her mom. They soon became an inseparable combination. At times you'd mistake them as an old husband and wife as they bickered and squabbled over the challenges of pre-teen issues.

At other times, they seemed to lean on each other for mutual support in a world of peer pressure, parents, and other day-to-day issues that worked to steer them in countless different directions as we entered the new millennium.

When elementary school faded into middle school, they were still there for each other. At a time when budding romances were occurring all around them, no such thing was in the cards for these two. Based on a mutual respect, theirs was a relationship few people their age ever contemplate. And so it went. John and Ashley critiquing other friends' relationships, playing football on the same middle school team (yes, football), going to dances, and generally gathering the same group around them as they made their way on to high school.

Ashley moved on to a private school in Rhode Island for high school. John would stay the local boy and attend his mom's alma-mater, Deering High School. The friendship remained through phone calls, e-mails, and weekend visits. It remains strong and binding. John reigned as champion in the battle against his hormones with Ashley. In the back of my mind, however, I think Ashley probably had more to do with that than John ever did. After all, he still has the Mallory gene.

22

Medi-Ports and Friends

Friends love misery, in fact. Sometimes, especially if we are too lucky or too successful or too pretty, our misery is the only thing that endears us to our friends.

~ Erica Jong

On October 24, John entered the Barbara Bush Wing of the Maine Medical Center in Portland, a facility that is well renowned for its care of children with childhood cancers. Because John was seventeen and almost, but not quite, an adult, the doctors decided that the best care for John would come from this facility.

John would receive a medi-port today. This device would serve as the entrance point for all medications delivered by needle. Implanted under his skin on the left side of his chest just above the heart, this round object protruded above the surface of the chest. Doctors explained to us that it would save the trouble of using veins, which were not ideal for chemo treatments. A tube ran from the port into a major vein. While the insertion was not a major operation, John would still require anesthesia for the second time in less than a week. Dr. Mallory would do the surgery and had explained it thoroughly to us days prior. (The coincidence of his name was not lost on us, and we tried to find any amusement in this juggernaut that was now running at full steam.)

Procedures that included a bone marrow biopsy, a full-body CT scan, and a pulmonary test also were scheduled to be performed. John's first chemo treatment would occur later that evening. The bone marrow biopsy and CT scan were to determine if John's lymphoma had spread to his bones and major organs below the chest. Chest X-rays and blood tests concluded the day's events.

This would not be an easy day for John. His second hospital experience was starting with a crash course in patience, boredom, and seemingly endless visits from nurses taking vital signs. He would need all his strength for his first chemo treatment later that day, but nothing they had done so far had led in that direction.

As I wound my way through a series of endless corridors and elevators to John's room, it struck me odd that, at this time of day, there seemed to be a flight of staff from the hospital. The late afternoon hour must have brought on a shift change, and I marveled at how these people, after dealing with pain and suffering all day, could simply turn it off and proceed home to make dinner. What strength of purpose medical professionals must have to make them want to do this type of work. Then I thought to myself, *Do all the good staff members works days? Who's going to be left here?*

I quickly found John's room where Nancy and Amanda were doting over John as he sat up in his hospital bed attached to an IV.

"Hey, Dad, want to see my medi-port?"

"Hi, John, how are you feeling? You okay?"

"Come on, let me show you."

"Fine, show me please, John."

"Nice. Does it hurt to have it in?"

"Nah, they gave me stuff for the pain."

Perhaps it was his way of dealing with it, but he seemed so casual about the whole thing. To John, his new medi-port seemed a badge of honor rather than a device that would be used in the life-saving process he was about to begin. He carried on as if every seventeen-year-old boy would experience this sooner or later—until our first setback.

Cancer, "Okay."

Lymph node biopsy, "Whatever."

Survival rates, "Kewl."

Second operation and stuck in the hospital again, "They're really pissing me off, Dad. They won't let me eat!"

Adding to John's displeasure on this day was the fact that they wouldn't let him eat anything. Having last eaten the night before at eight, John was famished. The CT scan was scheduled for 6:00 PM.

John would not be allowed to eat until after it was completed. So here he was, twenty-two hours without food for someone who normally would eat regularly on the hour all day long. Our human food vacuum was being tortured in a manner that now started making him … well, shall we say a bit at odds with the whole process?

John then took the opportunity to start ragging on his friends. Where were they? Why hadn't they come to see him? Disappointment filled his eyes, and sarcasm shaded his voice as we three attendants just would not suffice at this moment. The bond had been broken, and that was all that mattered. They were his buds, the group whose goofy antics he readily joined, and the group who meant something to him in this time of need. Friendship, it seemed, had a clearer meaning for John this night as he continued ranting about the lack of food, the crummy television, and the fact he would miss yet another Friday night out.

I felt like calling his friends and inquiring, "What gives, guys?" But I didn't. It wasn't my place, and John would be mad if I did. I knew this had to play itself out, and responded to John by arguing in their defense that they were probably just scared—scared of what was happening to him, perhaps scared of the hospital, and scared that the thought of the teenage myth of indestructibility had finally been shattered.

In short order, in they all strolled—seven tall, handsome, gangly, goofy teenage boys with only one reason for being there. All stood there looking at their feet after having hailed John in familiar yet hushed tones:

"Dude."

"Hey, dude."

"Hey, what's up, dude?"

"How are you doing, dude?"

These were not the friends of John's I had seen a thousand times acting like typical teenage boys. These were friends who didn't know how to respond or what to say to what they were witnessing. The tough teen persona had melted away to a reality check that spoke volumes about who they really were, how much they cared, and what this moment really meant to them.

John sensed it I believe. His smile was a mile wide as he quickly started pointing out his tubes, showing off his medi-port, and explaining the bed. Nancy and I sat back and breathed a collective sigh of relief as the room quickly filled with the same lame comments and observations I had heard from this group of big lugs so many times before. They were at ease with themselves now. If John could brush it off, so could they. If John could suck it up and play the tough teen, then they would also.

John made both of us very proud that evening. With all the indignities of the day, the pain we knew was there, and the thoughts of things to come later, John rose above it to make his friends feel comfortable and wanted. In the few short days since this nightmare had started, he had elevated himself to a different persona. The transformation from "teen-age John" to "young man John" had begun.

For rationales I don't remember, the CT scan was postponed. They later postponed it a second time. At 9:30 that evening, after twenty-five and a half hours without food of any kind, John was finely allowed a hospital meal. It goes without saying that, when I asked him later if the meal was any good, "teen-age John" simply responded, "It sucked, Dad, really sucked."

23

Learning an Art

By perseverance the snail reached the ark.

~ Charles Haddon Spurgeon

Many parents fall prey to the mistaken belief that you can keep a child busy every moment of every day. "Idle hands are the devils plaything," so to speak. Play a sport, volunteer for this, what about a club at school? As time goes by, you also come to understand that everything they become interested in also requires you to drive them to and from wherever it's happening. Get them too interested in things, and it will take both of you to untangle your schedules to find a way to manage.

John was no different in this regard. One of the burgeoning sports in America today for young people is martial arts. Martial arts, it seems, exist in as many forms as there are automobile models, each defined by something that makes it different from all other forms. Introduced to jujitsu at the very impressionable age of seven, John became involved fast. After a few classes, a bond soon developed between him and his teacher.

Martial arts are not just a sport. Martial arts are a discipline, an art form, and a way of life for those serious about them. Everyone, age notwithstanding, starts at the same level. While you may be bigger and stronger at age twenty-one than you are at seven, your knowledge of the discipline grows equally. It was not uncommon to see a twelve-year-old John practicing with a room full of adults.

As John progressed through the many levels, we became acutely aware that this sport taught so much more than a physical activity.

When the instructor, called the sensei, speaks, the students listen. A routine that the sensei asked to be repeated over and over again was done out of respect for him and for the discipline. Inside the school—the dojo—students put aside all the antics of youth in favor of gaining the knowledge of the sensei. John grew both physically and mentally through the progressive belts, each of which signified an advance in his achievement. With only the occasional complaint about missing this or that, he faithfully attended every session, testing for every level and moving forward until the big day arrived.

Achieving any level of black belt in the martial arts is a testament to the individual receiving the honor. John's prize was attainable when he reached the age of fourteen, after seven years of study. He had created lasting friendships with a group of people—mostly adults—who had also worked hard to reach this level. He'd stuck with it and gained the respect of his peers, his sensei, and his parents. What had started out as something to keep John busy in his spare time now ended with the award he coveted so badly.

Bravo! Bravo John Mallory!

24

Chemotherapy

Everything is a dangerous drug except reality, which is unendurable.
~ Cyril Connolly

In countless numbers of research facilities around the world, a collection of geniuses works tirelessly to solve the mysteries of cancer. Perhaps it was their first chemistry set they received one Christmas, perhaps curiosity, or perhaps these pioneers find it infinitely more rewarding to try to find cures than to chase the almighty dollar and be rewarded with a seven-figure income and an early coronary. Whatever the reason, these dedicated heroes have given millions of people afflicted with the insidious nature of cancer the hope of survival. It is this hope that carried us into John's first "chemo" session.

Chemotherapy is the systematic administration of a combination of medicines, a recipe if you will. Each patient receives a different recipe based on what he or she is facing. For John, the first treatment would be a combination of five different medicines injected into his mediport. As I understood it, the immune system had failed to do its job of preventing the lymphoma, so the chemo medicines say, "Okay, fella, take a break; we're taking over."

The medicines all have names with at least fifteen letters that the best English teacher would have a hard time pronouncing. The name of one medicine, however, I will never forget: nitrogen mustard. In this first round of chemo, we would become all too familiar with this drug. If the name sounds familiar, it's because this drug has some of the same properties that are found in mustard gas, the chemical warfare agent used first against troops in the First World War. If it comes in contact with the skin, it burns. When it is administered in chemotherapy, staff members suit up accordingly. Go figure.

John's first experience with this drug and the four others he received the first time was not pleasant. Nancy got but little sleep this first night in the hospital as she stood guard over John like a Roman sentry. If he needed anything, she was there. At four thirty, the vomiting started, and John gave up the hospital meal he had as much as begged for only hours before.

The next three days at home produced extreme bouts of nausea followed by vomiting, more nausea, and a terrible fatigue. John looked as bad as he felt. As he moved from his bed to the couch and back again, Nancy tried in vain to get him to eat something. White rice and a few crackers would be her only victories, but it was a start. John looked for all the world like a Holocaust survivor. With sunken cheeks and a grayish color, he'd drag his comforter around walking aimlessly throughout the house trying to fight the nausea that kept returning.

Just a week earlier, John and Amanda had been enjoying each other at Homecoming. It seemed so long ago. Now he was in the battle of his young life. I thought to myself, *Can he handle it? Will it overwhelm him? Is his skinny little body capable of fighting for him? Will all the treatments be this bad?* All the questions swirled about, never stopping, and more questions came as the days went on.

John fought through those first days and made us keenly aware of how he would keep fighting. I saw courage in him that I had never seen before. I saw a stalwart attitude that forecast how he would deal with this disease. He knew the alternatives, and he kept focused in a manner that would not let him dwell on it, at least outwardly. He had him mom, his dad, and he had Amanda. He understood one thing: We'd work together as a team to get him better.

25

Stupid Is as Stupid Does

Character cannot be developed in ease and quiet. Only through experience of trial and suffering can the soul be strengthened, ambition inspired, and success achieved.

~ Helen Keller

First, let me make one thing perfectly clear. I don't condone underage drinking or illegal drug use. Having grown up in the '60s, I know all too well the negative impact both can have on an individual, especially for someone whose brain is competing to soak up knowledge at the same time.

Fast forward to the year 2008, the new millennium, and the X generation. Drugs have made their way into the mainstream lives of a significant portion of today's young people. While the young people of Portland, Maine, and Deering High School in particular are no exception, it surprised me to know that John was among them. We had preached for a significant portion of John's young life about the downside of drugs and alcohol, but as early as the later years of middle school, the signs were there that John was experimenting.

I think we fought the good fight, always taking an opportunity to preach the gospel of college, illegality, and brain cell loss. We lost the fight ultimately to friends and peer pressure, the scourge of any parent. We could scream and holler, we could ground him, we could take away computers, cell phones, television, and car privileges—and ultimately nothing worked. The rebellion was running its course. The best we could hope for was that, ultimately, John would make the right choices. Were we bad parents? Did we give up too easily? Would John fall into a depravity because of his "reefer madness?"

John got good grades and participated in all honors and advanced placement (AP) classes. He never got behind the wheel when he shouldn't have. He loved his parents and was polite. How could we argue with this?

But we did, right up until the night his friends delivered John on our doorstep so intoxicated he couldn't walk or talk. The results of drinking a pint of Knob Creek in a very short amount of time were astonishing to witness. We were scared to death, thinking we should call an ambulance and get him to the hospital. We showered him, and, after he vomited several times, we thought it safe enough to put him to bed, where Nancy kept vigil the entire night.

Over the ensuing months, we argued, urged, threatened, and cajoled until the morning at work I got a call from John telling me he had been caught smoking pot on school property. With me being a school employee—someone whose kid should set an example—we were again caught in the cross fire. This time was different, though. This time, the full weight of the justice system would fall on John. Maybe it was just what he needed. Maybe this would shake some sense into him.

"Do you want a record?" I asked.

"No."

"Do you want to go to college, John?"

"Yes."

"Then do me a favor for once and get with the program. There are a million kids just like you handing out burgers at McDonalds from coast to coast. That could be you."

"I know."

And so it went, each success followed by a new failure. I'm not sure what hurt most, the self-destructive nature of what he was doing, or the fact that he defied us so often. He knew that, in 2008, it wasn't easy to get lucky and get a break that would later help you rise up the ladder. He knew that, for every kid who graduated college, there were just as many languishing in unemployment lines. Yet it continued, culminating in the last event that was the proverbial "straw that broke the camel's back" for Nancy and I, and. I think, in many ways, for him also.

It seems the newest entrepreneurial offering at high school in the winter of 2008 was to acquire alcohol, put it in drink containers that camouflaged its identity, and sell it at school. I don't fault the school. I mean, who knew? Until these "business people" started getting caught. And caught was what John was. It could have been when he threw up in French class, but more likely it was when he chose to attend swimming practice after school at a pool where it had to be one hundred degrees. Out came the breathalyzer, and off went John, banished from the swim team.

John liked swimming and had spent the better part of his young life taking lessons and competing. He was getting good, and we looked forward to a year where things would start paying off for him in the pool. It was not to be. To his credit, John made the appropriate apologies and started moving in a different direction. This one had hurt, probably more so than anything Nancy and I had said in the past. He had lost something he liked doing, and I'm sure he was asking himself, *Was it worth it?* Of course not. It was a dumb ass thing to do, and he knew it. It was "punk" as the kids say. It was "stupid is as stupid does" as Forest Gump would say.

This was not a life-defining moment. It did leave John with an understanding of how people viewed people who continue to do dumb things. John was not dumb by any stretch of the imagination. He knew he was better than that. He'd have to prove it to himself somehow, and, in the months ahead, somehow we knew he would.

26

Riding the Waves

Tomorrow is the most important thing in life. Comes into us at midnight very clean. It's perfect when it arrives and it puts itself in our hands. It hopes we've learned something from yesterday.

~ John Wayne

Live in Maine, and you'll soon discover there are two months that hold a dreariness to match no other. November crosses over between fall and winter, and April crosses over between spring and summer. In November, high gray clouds usher in the cold, and you mutter, "Oh damn, it's almost here." In April, short-lived bursts of warmth tease the mind, and you mutter, "Oh yay, it's almost here!" And so it was that November—cold, dreary, and unbending in its trek toward winter.

The nausea that feasted on John's body during his early treatments had subsided thanks to more medical miracles, this time coming in the form of an IV that kept the demons at rest for seven days at a time. Along with his other nausea meds, John was managing to rebound quicker after every treatment.

We soon settled into a pattern that brought the nurse to our home on Mondays to draw blood for the lab work that was necessary before the next chemo treatment, which happened on Wednesdays. The nurses were a godsend, saving us from having to travel to the cancer center, or trying to do the unthinkable, draw blood ourselves. Each week, Nancy would hover over the nurses instructing them on which needle to use and asking questions. To the nurses, she was probably being a general pain in the ass. They never seemed to act that way, however, as I know they deemed this a mother's duty, a duty that Nancy responded to with a "don't mess with me" look in her eyes each time a nurse would open a fresh needle.

For his part, John would sit quietly on a kitchen stool, stripped to his waist and patiently waiting for the routine to continue so he could get back to whatever it was he had been doing. This was just another interruption to tolerate, just another piece of the progress path he was forced to endure. John had become almost robotic in his response to the whole process.

The wave would arrive on Wednesday. We never knew what to expect afterward. Fatigue was what plagued John the most, that and the increasing amount of pain after each treatment. His bones and muscles all hurt in response to the chemo. At times walking like an old man, John would simply flop on the couch and quietly moan.

Of course, there was a pill for that. I don't know many of the names, but there were pills for nausea, heavy duty drugs for pain, pills to stimulate the appetite, drugs to make him go to the bathroom, and other pill bottles lining the kitchen counter whose purpose was probably only known to Nancy. So many pills that she took to using a pillbox for each day with sections marked, "morning," "noon," and "evening." She knew all the drugs by name, knew the importance of each, and, for better or worse, she keenly remained aware of each medicine's side effects.

School was a challenge to say the least. John's attendance was built around his treatment schedule. On Mondays and Tuesdays, John found the energy to attend a limited amount of school, but often would leave after a couple of hours because of fatigue and the resulting inability to focus. On Wednesdays, he'd squeeze in a half day before his treatment. And Thursdays and Fridays were more or less a guessing game. The teachers and the school were great in the makeup work department, so much so that John managed to complete the first semester of his junior year with one A and three Bs.

And so, on it went, one wave after another, each one taking John one step closer to ridding himself of this interruption in his life ... one step closer to moving toward a normalcy that was John's comfort zone. He didn't complain; he did what he had to do. We all did.

27

New Freedoms

The best way to keep children home is to make the home atmosphere pleasant—and let the air out of the tires.

~ Dorothy Parker

A driver's license is the first true ticket to freedom that is bestowed on a teenager. Mobility and the ability to travel freely beyond the neighborhood is truly a precious commodity. No more "take me here, take me there." A driver's license is the bridge to adulthood, the ultimate move to being "kewl."

When I was growing up, a license was out of my reach. It cost money to drive a car—money my parents didn't have. And I could never have accumulated enough money to buy a vehicle on my own. There was always someone with a license, though, someone willing to drag my sorry butt along for the ride. That was enough for me. Inconvenient yes, but cheap also.

John, of course, being a child of the new millennium, would have none of that. He had to be the first one on the block to "bag his plastic." And, of course, Nancy and I went along not wanting John to be "unkewl." We had no choice; the incessant badgering started at fourteen and ran unabated for months until it was time for him to take his driver's training. We were beaten. And for a mother who had managed every aspect of John's life by cell phone when he was away from home, that was not a good thing.

Drivers training soon led to The Test. We've all been there. Here he was, the grumpy state worker who would rather have been anywhere else than taking his life into his own hands when putting these neophyte drivers through *his* prearranged course. If you were going to get your license, you'd get it on his terms. He'd find the railroad tracks, the stop signs, the right-on-red traffic lights, the divided highways, and any other number of pitfalls designed to test even the most experienced driver.

With a confidence built from many accompanied hours behind the wheel, John strode off to do battle. In his mind, he couldn't fail. To him, failure was out of the question. Failure was for his buddies, but not for him. Well, he failed.

Mad? Yup.

Ticked off? Oh yeah!

Defeated? Nope, not the slightest chance he'd fail again.

This was John. He'd pick up the pieces and we'd pay another fee to get him behind the wheel. Only this time, he knew the game. Grumpy guy would not win.

As he proudly announced his accomplishment to me over the phone, I thought to myself, *Well, here we go, the next act is about to begin.*

That night, John took the car for the first time by himself. His cry of freedom rang loud and clear.

28

Faith

Faith and religion, of course, are not one and the same. The distinction between the two is similar to the distinction between what is sometimes referred to as the soul and body of an experience. The soul is the invisible part, rooted in the mind, will, and feelings. The body of the experience is the outward expression of its soul. It is the putting into action of an idea, conviction, hope or desire. Faith, then, is like the soul of an experience. It is an inner acknowledgment of the relationship between God and man. Religion, on the other hand, is like the body. It is an outer expression of that inner acknowledgment.

~ John Powell

As the days dragged slowly toward Thanksgiving, the cards, e-mails, and phone calls soon outstripped our ability to thank everyone individually in a timely fashion. I took to e-mailing people in a group to keep them updated, something I thought was a bit tacky to say the least, but nonetheless effective.

Food, flowers, and small gifts were keeping Nancy busy with thank-you cards, and John supplied with an endless supply of junk food. Say what you will, the junk food kept his weight up. If he wouldn't eat a stir-fry, he would at least munch endless bags of chips. It didn't matter; he was eating.

Through the cards and e-mails, we became aware that friends whom we never thought were terribly religious were offering prayers for John. Along those same lines, others would simply state that their "thoughts were with us." Aha! Now we could tell who the true heathens were among us.

Include myself in this group. Put through our paces by old-school Catholic parents, obligations made were obligations met. Mass on Sunday, mass for Holy Days of Obligation, mass for weddings, mass for funerals, and mass on every day of Holy Week, it seemed that the religion wanted us constantly in church where they could keep an eye on us. Then there was catechism, the church's idea of Saturday torture where we actually attended school and learned how to be a good Catholic. Okay already, we had learned about faith, believed in Jesus Christ, and had found our savior. Enough already, you made your point!

I'm not at all sure when it started—probably about the time I left home and struck out on my own—but the idea of formal religion just didn't excite me. I was a believer, and I thought of myself as a good person. But, what did worshiping in a building have to do with finding eternal salvation?

I didn't believe in the church's doctrines concerning abortion, gays, or priests marrying. The church seemed so old fashioned. My liberal leanings had me thinking this was not a church for everyone. I gave in anyway, more to appease the traditionalists than for any other reason. We had John baptized. Nancy and I were also remarried in the church after annulments of my previous two marriages (fifty bucks apiece); a compatibility test (after five years of marriage we flunked it); and, last but not least, confession. I found myself sitting across from a Franciscan monk trying to explain to him all the tawdry things I had done in the past thirty years. Shivers ran up my spine as I held back more than I told him. Nancy met the same fate.

It was with this backdrop that Nancy and I decided that, if John wanted religion, he'd find it on his own. We'd let him decide what was right for him and not make him follow in our footsteps. For better or worse and against all our teachings, he was on his own to make choices about whom and what he wanted to be. John would find faith at some point in his life if he chose to.

As the prayers kept pouring in from our friends, family members, and co-workers, I couldn't bring myself to ask for anything from the big guy. I felt as if I had temporarily ditched my faith for years, and to ask now would be most hypocritical on my part. I have never questioned him as to why we have experienced all of the recent turmoil. If there is a reason, and I believe there has to be, it will show its face at some point.

It's often said that faith can move mountains. My faith, though battered and bruised recently, is still intact. Thank you, Jesus.

29

Thanksgiving

The reason grandparents and grandchildren get along so well is that they have a common enemy.

~Sam Levenson

As Thanksgiving approached, Nancy and I put our plan together for feeding the eleven people who would be coming to dinner. Gourmet that she is, in the past when we hosted, everything had to be just so. With the world spinning out of control this year, and having made the plans before John was diagnosed, our main focus seemed to be more of, "let's just get it over with, and hope the turkey isn't dry."

John awoke Thanksgiving morning looking and sounding like someone had worked him over in a title bout. He body ached all over, his stomach was bothering him, and he shuffled along like an old man. Even on Thanksgiving, there was no respite from the sixth chemo he had received the day before. As we went through the paces of final meal preparations, John mounted enough energy to somehow go off and pick up Amanda. If only for a couple of hours, John's rock would be where he wanted her most.

Extended families and major holidays create choices each year that often pull us in different directions. For Nancy, it was easier than most. Her ninety-three-year-old father, wandering the world of dementia, always went with his wife to her son's for Thanksgiving. We respected this tradition and felt that "Daddy" honored his wife by participated yearly. With Nancy's only sister living in Massachusetts, we would make our yearly choices of friends or family on Thanksgiving, but always left

Christmas set aside for the Mallory clan. It was no different this year with one brother opting to be with friends, one brother opting to be with a wife whose brother was himself battling cancer, and another brother whose wife was sick staying home for fear of passing something on to John. It was a most welcome group that joined us on this sobering Thanksgiving.

My mom and dad, eighty-nine and eighty-two respectively, greeted us, but, even with the worldliness of their years, they found it tough to greet and hug John. I thought back to the boys in the hospital and watched as John hugged them and tried to make them feel at ease. There wasn't much said between them; there didn't have to be.

John's hair had been falling out now, and he'd been in the habit of pulling out small pieces, so his scalp resembled a dotted cue ball. Even he knew it looked bad. His solution? Shave it bald. It was going in that direction anyway; at least it would all look the same. With the two of them bickering like an old couple after years and years of marriage, Amanda shaved his nearly bald scalp clean that night before Thanksgiving.

John surprised me. I had thought that he would bare his newly shaved head to show everyone that it wasn't any big deal to lose your hair from cancer treatments. He didn't, though. He wore his bandana as if to say, "don't focus on me, have fun, I'm okay."

That's just what happened. No one focused on John. They focused on being together as a family as we had always done in the past. We were there for him, just as we were for each other.

30

Kayaks

A life on the ocean wave
A home on the rolling deep
Where the scattered waters rave
And the winds their revels keep!
Like an eagle caged I pine
On this dull unchanging shore:
Oh give me the flashing brine,
The spray and the tempest's roar!

~ Epes Sargent

Brought up within a mile of the coastline, I took the ocean very much for granted. I saw it every day, but rarely took the opportunity to discover its unique majesty. In South Portland, the proximity of the shore allowed the neighborhood guys to go crabbing and fishing off the rickety piers that once had been the city's lifeblood. Willard Beach, the forts, the lighthouses—all seemed so ordinary to us. We didn't see these places as grandiose the way a Midwesterner would; we saw them as places to hang out and have fun.

With our never-ending quest to find something for John to do in the summer, Nancy found Ripple Effect, a nonprofit organization that specializes in training young people to handle kayaks and learn leadership skills in combination with being good stewards of the environment. John and Ripple Effect clicked immediately.

Early on, John showed a talent with the small craft. He mastered them quickly and enjoyed being on the water, even though they wouldn't venture far from shore the first years. As he progressed, he learned kayak rolls, leadership, safety, and a respect for the environment of Casco Bay. With each new summer, John became more and more adept at the adventures fashioned for his age group.

My dad was a lobsterman. Fresh out of World War II, he saw this as a means of not only feeding a growing family, but a way to be independent and a way to enjoy his first love, the sea. It goes without saying that Dad exposed us to his way of life by occasionally taking my older brother and me on board for the day. Standing flat footed next to him in a small, open boat as we hauled traps in rough seas is one lasting memory I have of my Dad. Jumping onto the nearest piece of land in sea-sick agony is my lasting memory of the sea. For obvious reasons, I never appreciated lobster fishing or being that close to the sea; for John it was a magnet.

John's unique opportunity to kayak the coast of Maine made each summer an event. The goal of the group was to pick a different sector of the coast that they could adventure on for a one-week period. I cringed at the thought of John in a sea kayak on the open ocean. For Nancy, it was pins and needles all the way. Were they taking care of him? Was he getting enough to eat? What about the guides—were they qualified enough? With each passing day he spent on the water, she managed to hold it together enough without cell phone contact until the final day when he showed up on the dock beaming his approval of his just completed "man adventure."

We very much welcomed his last trip as a time when we could relax and enjoy the fact that no crisis would occur for a week of our summer. John was off to explore the costal area of Castine, Maine, with the same enthusiasm and gusto he'd displayed for prior trips. As we settled into our quiet week, it soon became apparent it would be anything but.

A ringing phone late one evening duly informed us that John had sustained an injury trying to prove his manhood by scaling a cliff on the island they were exploring. All hell had immediately broken loose. A lobster boat had conveyed John back to the mainland, and a waiting ambulance had whisked him off to Blue Hill Hospital. Stitched up and none the worse for wear, he had spent the night at the home of a local woman volunteer. At dawn (actually a few hours earlier), Nancy bolted to retrieve him. Super Mom was off to the rescue.

I've often thought that John's time on the sea shaped the person he was turning into. He has a deep respect for the ocean and what it means to be miles from shore with just the training he has received. There is no fear of what it means to be paddling in the fog with just a compass. He also learned quickly that the ocean and its reach can just swallow him up if he doesn't respect its awesome power.

The ever-changing sea was good to John, and he to it.

31

Medicinal Use Only

Behind every argument is someone's ignorance.

~ Louis D. Brandeis

There is a medicine whose trade name is Marinol. It resembles a tiny, clear gumball. You have to keep it refrigerated. One of the active ingredients in this drug is THC. Correct … the same compound found in marijuana. With a prescription, it is legal to purchase Marinol in the United States. For cancer patients, it increases the appetite and helps with nausea.

When John—I should say his parents—let the doctors know that he was a casual pot smoker, they explained to him that, because his lungs had to be working at top capacity, and because they didn't really know what is actually in marijuana, they would like him to refrain from using it, and to use the Marinol instead. Before she could finish, John was on the bandwagon. Just as quickly, he slumped back in his seat when the doctor explained there was no high associated with this drug. Easy come, easy go.

Our focus from the start was always to make John as comfortable as possible, to make sure he ate, to keep the nausea at bay, and to make sure he got his meds when scheduled. We hadn't been warned much about the pain and fatigue. The only thing that was mentioned was that some people experienced different levels of each with the treatments.

John took the Marinol occasionally, and he remarked that it made him really hungry when he took it. Really hungry, of course, meant that, in most cases, he would rarely eat more than half of the food put in front of him. It did nothing for the pain. For the pain, we were left to the oxy family of drugs; these heavyweights would have to do the trick.

They did work to a certain extent, but we feared dependency as we heard many horror stories about these drugs. Even though John's chances of becoming dependent were slim, we still used them sparingly. Nancy ended up hiding them when we discovered John felt the need to self-medicate.

In every state, it is illegal to grow or purchase marijuana for recreational use. In a few places, it may be grown and sold for medicinal purposes only. Maine has a law on the books, but doctors will still not accommodate prescriptions. Early on, Nancy and I made a pact. Based on John's past, we would not succumb to allowing John to smoke marijuana. Exercising all other options came first.

We soon gave in when it was apparent that his medications weren't helping with his stomach issues or the pain as they should have been. I don't know if John was being sincere, or if it really worked to suppress the pain and make him feel better, as he said it did. It didn't matter. Legality could take a backseat for now if he felt better.

At the first sign of remission, we planned to ground John for a year.

32

High School

High school wasn't a trial by fire or some ordeal that had to be survived. It was all a big joke. You just had to provide the laugh track.

~ Scott Westerfeld

John has never recorded anything but As and Bs on his report card through this his junior year of high school. With all the outside influences that press at teenagers these days, this remarkable feat stands in stark contrast to the amount of work he actually does to achieve these grades.

High school is John's playground. In a school of over eleven hundred students, with the exception of a few I'm sure, he seems to be everyone's friend, or least an acquaintance. While his core group has remained intact, he's captured more and more friends as the years have passed.

John goes through the motions of high school as if it's just something to tolerate on his way to the "big show," whatever he thinks that might be. His study habits are terrible, his work ethic nonexistent, and never (well almost never) has he gone to the extent of doing extra credit work. Without our continual badgering, homework would be a lost cause.

Forget about clubs or activities. He wouldn't raise a finger to get involved in any of them, even though his parents have remarked constantly that involvement will surely help when college administrators weed out the deadwood.

His classes are all honors courses sprinkled with an advanced placement course here or there. He moans about still taking French, having studied it since the third grade, but he is close to becoming fluent at the same time. He loves history, and takes after me in that regard.

While college is a definite in his future, he approaches it as he approaches everything else. With an attitude of "we'll face it only when we need to," he has done nothing to get himself interested. He doesn't express an interest in talking about "majors" and is only willing to declare that working in the outdoors is in his future.

So let's recap. Good grades, advanced classes, plenty of friends, knows a language, and, oh, one other thing, his parents will be footing the entire bill for college!

I just don't get it. He has so much going for him. If I had been in his position at his age, I might have turned out to be a doctor, lawyer, or Indian chief somewhere with a hefty six-figure income. What does it take to motivate these days? Are parents supposed to motivate through their vision of their future? Or are kids supposed to motivate themselves through their own vision?

Recently John has missed a lot of school. He tires easily and has to come home. Many days he feels terrible in the morning and has a difficult time getting out of bed. We are always in a quandary. Do we tell him to suck it up, or just leave him alone?

He has made up his backlog of work from the first semester half, and now we are pushing into the second half. I've left him alone, much to his mom's chagrin, and figure it just isn't all that important right now. I can't even imagine what it must be like for him, having what he has hanging over his head as the physics teacher trudges through Newton's Law. If it takes more time to finish high school, so be it.

I'm going to let him sleep tomorrow. He looks terrible, mostly because I goaded him into going to school all day today. It's not my life, it's his. I'm being terribly unfair. If he wants to sit back and be Jimmy Buffet the rest of his life, he's earned it.

33

Middle Age Put on Hold

The only time you really live fully is from thirty to sixty. The young are slaves to dreams; the old servants of regrets. Only the middle-aged have all their five senses in the keeping of their wits.

~ Hervey Allen

We all seem to know roughly when middle age starts, but most assuredly refuse to accept when it ends. It comes on in stages, and somewhere between our past experiences and the unknowns of the future, it hits us squarely between the eyes: we're getting old.

The anxieties of wanting to play a good round of golf to impress friends slowly give way to the hope we'll have enough golf balls left in the bag to finish the round. At the moment we least expect it, middle age engulfs us firmly in its grasp. We understand where we are headed. With the last of the golf balls gone and few, if any, good shots left to impress friends, we quietly morph into someone more receptive to unabashedly declaring, "What the hell, let's skip the back nine, enjoy the scenery on the way back, and just have lunch."

We were ready to accept the predictability of middle age as nothing more than a springboard to the green pastures of retirement. Nancy and I didn't challenge middle age, or embrace it. Nor did we purchase any new golf clubs.

The idea of advanced middle age held a certain allure. For myself at least, I reasoned that it was inescapable and welcome—a part-time job to keep busy ("paper or plastic?"), warm summer days at the lake, and making sure the four o'clock cocktail was more for the pleasure of it than for the medicinal value it offered.

Of course, the fleeting thoughts of a parent's mortality paled in comparison to the issues we were now facing. It didn't matter. Our lives, for better or worse, were now on hold. Cancer had done that as surely as if someone had put a brick wall directly in our path.

Middle age came with the slow predictability we had hoped for. Sprinkled sometimes with doubts, mind-numbing challenges, and an overabundance of question, it nonetheless held up to its billing.

For every success—the paying off of a mortgage, a raise, a new automobile—there was a leaking pipe, a roof needing replacement, or a retirement account dwindling away. We shrugged, mustered enough energy to deal with the current issue, and moved on. It never tore at us, it was what it was: life. It seemed predictable and plausible.

But, cancer presented itself as something ludicrous. We had taken everything life had thrown at us from all angles and managed each event successfully, but this new challenge left us decidedly confused, wounded, and feeling as if the past meant little now.

John's cancer was a wake-up call. We'd been too complacent and lost in day-to-day outcomes to even consider anything of such a horrible nature befalling us. His cancer made it clear to us that, as predictable as life seems, as well planned out your notion of the future is, and as sheltered as you think you are from the evils from the outside, another test is always lurking around the corner.

How did the predictability of the arrival of middle age slowly grind to a halt after so many years? I don't know, but it happened—middle age and the security we believed would come with it had suddenly stuck its finger in our face and reminded us, "You got a ways to go yet, folks."

34

Wednesdays

A hero is someone who rebels or seems to rebel against the facts of existence and seems to conquer them. Obviously that can only work at moments. It can't be a lasting thing. That's not saying that people shouldn't keep trying to rebel against the facts of existence. Someday, who knows, we might conquer death, disease and war.

~ Jim Morrrison

Lovingly referred to by the working world as "hump day," Wednesday is the day when you start to see the light at the end of the tunnel and breathe a sigh of relief that soon you'll have two days without the daily pressures that pound at us relentlessly.

Wednesdays now held a new meaning for us. Wednesday was chemo day. This was the day that John would receive the mind-boggling concoctions that would bring him down the road of recovery. Wednesday, a day loathed by all of us, came all too soon each week. We knew that relief from the side effects occurred in the earlier part of the week. We knew that the end of the week would bring difficult days.

Nancy always handled the chemo sessions. To her, it became an unthinkable notion that I escort John to these sessions for fear that I would forget to write down something important the doctors said or forget to ask an important question. This was, in all likelihood, a smart move on her part, but nonetheless the duty was becoming as debilitating for her as it was for John.

Depending on the different types of drugs pumped into John, Wednesdays became predictable to a certain extent. There were milder drugs, all the way up to the five-drug cocktail, which we referred to with much disdain as "the mustard." It was all marked out for us in "the schedule" that some scientist somewhere had laid out for this particular disease as the best possible course of treatment.

Each visit brought the same routine: the weigh-in, the blood count results, the needles, and so on. There wasn't much to decipher from these sessions. The real telling would come later from the CT scan, the PET scan, and the pulmonary scan, all of which would occur in December and give us the first real chance to see if the chemo was doing its job properly.

John has three small tumors in his right lung, a tumor on his neck, and a massive tumor near his right lung. This was the "Big Boy" as I referred to it. "Big Boy" caused problems because it actually displaced things in his chest. It was our primary concern and the main focus for us as we looked ahead to the tests.

When God calls the employees of The Maine Children's Cancer to heaven, they won't have to wait at the gates. They will be ushered in and surely sit at his right hand, no questions asked. It is a remarkable person who can deal with this kind of pain and suffering on a daily basis with children—and their parents. The grace and guidance they have bestowed on us each Wednesday during this process have made the sessions and their aftermath bearable. Their understanding and patience go far beyond human kindness. They are true heroes.

35

Donuts and Fuzzy Bears

The ideals which have lighted my way, and time after time have given me new courage to face life cheerfully, have been kindness, beauty, and truth. The trite subjects of human efforts, possessions, outward success, and luxury have always seemed to me contemptible.

~ Albert Einstein

There is always someone who goes above and beyond in situations like John's that make it all seem that much more bearable. Such was the case with Dan Lucas and Auntie Kaye Mallory. I don't think they ever met each other; it doesn't matter. What matters is that they both responded to John in a manner that said, "Don't you worry one second, Johnny, someone is always going to be there when the chips are down."

For Dan, it was donuts. Not just any donuts, but Tony's Donuts.

I've never been a fan of these donuts, but to Dan and John they were heavenly delights. They were food that you could stuff down your gullet two or three at a time and wash down with a cold glass of milk. This was food you could eat anytime—morning, noon, or night. This was junk food with a capital *J*.

Dan would deliver John's ration two or three times a week by showing up at the front door early in the morning and proclaiming "donut delivery!" It was Dan's personal mission to fatten up the patient even if he had to do it with some of the unhealthiest food on the planet. He knew John would succumb at some point and start pounding the monsters. The fat transfer from donuts to John would soon accomplish Dan's goal and bring the piggy boy out of his shell.

John did not disappoint. He did his part to keep Tony's Donut Shop thriving, and to make sure that Dan's delivery was a most welcome event.

When Auntie Kaye announced that she was coming over with a gift she'd bought for John, I was thinking along the lines of a book, a CD, or possibly something John liked to eat. But, she strode into the living holding a stuffed bear whose expression was rather goofy. I thought to myself, *Oh, god, John, just be gracious and except it from the heart.*

What John did next floored us all. With a beaming smile a mile wide, he took the bear from Auntie Kaye and cuddled it close. Here he was, "Joe Kewl," the one teenager on the planet you never thought would react this way, responding the same way he had at Christmases past when Whinnie the Pooh jumped from the box.

It was a sight I will always remember. This stuffed bear with paws with claws had found a place in John's heart. He was not that far removed from being a child, and I think in some sense the bear brought back pleasant memories to him. The bear—I forget his name—has a permanent home on John's bed now.

Thank you, Auntie Kaye. Thank you, Dan. Thank you both for taking John's thoughts off the moment and back to simpler times.

Simple acts of kindness flowed during that November. People's hearts were broken over John's plight. They coped with their feelings and managed, time and again, to make the ordeal more tolerable for us as the low points continued to mount up. They'd show up in the nick of time for a drink, some conversation, or to drop off a complete dinner to relieve Nancy and I of the food prep task.

Friends and family solidified their bonds with us, always encouraging, patient, and understanding as they shared the journey with us, a journey that was as much theirs to them as it was ours to us. We weren't alone, and we felt it.

36

A Mountain in Maine

Although golf was originally restricted to wealthy, overweight Protestants, today it's open to anybody who owns hideous clothing.

Dave Barry

It's not difficult to become overwhelmed by the shear thought of your child having cancer. We tried not to talk about it much, somehow thinking in our minds that the less said the better. We focused on the day-to-day functions of the family, the appointments, and even school to a certain extent. We talked honestly about what was important to us. While laughter seemed in short supply, we always made a point to revisit in conversation past events and times to take our minds off the present. Nancy and I would sit and critique such past moments if for no other reason than to force ourselves to remember good times and to convince ourselves of their inevitable return.

The week before we received news about John's condition seemed in our minds so far away now. With our busy work schedules, we had never really rehashed The Great Mid-Life Golfing Event to any extent before the world of cancer consumed us. Yet, here in the midst of such overwhelming dread, we'd revisit events such as this in the hope that some solace would be forthcoming and that our sanity would remain intact. Remembering made us laugh and took away the hurt that all but consumed us.

Sugarloaf USA is a ski resort in western Maine. It is busy in the winter, and, save for a few conferences, sleepy at best during the summer. Fall is a different story. Breathtaking is what best describes this area.

We had planned a weekend getaway one night during the past summer, when the wine had taken over, and distance (two and half hours) was no object. My wife of twenty-two years and our friends Judy and Jack had looked forward to this outing as a time to just do "anything that falls our way." One round of golf on the world-famous Sugarloaf Golf Course was our only commitment. Our wedding anniversary and Nancy's birthday falling on this same weekend added to our expectations.

Beauty aside, there is another reason they call golf courses such as Sugarloaf "world famous." They are, to say at the very least, quite challenging to play for the average hacker. Did I say quite challenging? Maybe heartbreaking, demeaning, uncomfortable, tragic, and just a plain pain in the ass would better describe the beauty of this perfect piece of green.

Hack-and-whacks such as Nancy and I don't attempt courses of this magnitude; they just watch other people play them on television. People with low handicaps understand the meaning of the term "world famous." With a "we'll see" attitude and a determination that no golf course is *that* hard, they relish the idea of playing them with a special zeal. Such is Jack.

After a night of middle-age cavorting, that is to say, too much wine, and no common sense, we thrust ourselves into the crisp autumn air of a no-kids Saturday morning. Needless to say, no amount of fresh air would have an impact on the size of our heads, the dryness in our throats, or the ability of at least three of us to play anything that resembled the true game of golf.

When weekend golfers the likes of Nancy and me drive up to a golf club such as this in their friends' Mercedes, one can only marvel as the world stands still and the word *sir* jumps forth from the mouths of babes who know just what a Mercedes means. You guessed it—a bit fat tip. Not to disappoint, our traveling companion was more than ready to oblige. You see, middle age does come with its benefits. Lest I vent my venom on the new generation of entitled children, "Yes, Virginia, working your ass off does pay dividends." You work, you pay, you work some more, and pay some more, and one day you find yourself with a tire around your waist and a new bald spot, tipping the help and playing golf on a world-famous golf course.

As expected, we three unpracticed golfers did not disappoint. For my part, I proudly stepped to the first tee and launched the first two balls into the woods. My thoughts of trying to impress anyone stopped right there. The quest to finish with at least one ball left in my bag had begun.

As a seasoned golfer, Jack surveyed the first hole, and casually stated, "I'll try the gold tees and see what happens." Did he say gold? Fifty yards back from my tee box he swung the club as effortlessly as I knew he would. Long and straight, his ball soared into the autumn air, with the ranger applauding, "Great shot, you're in fine shape." Well at least one of us had his clear definition of middle age down pat. Long and straight was not in my vocabulary; for Jack, it fit perfectly.

Throughout the morning, without keeping score, we managed to get around the course. We savored a few good shots while cringing at a multitude of disappointing ones. We managed to finally relax, enjoy the scenery, and accept the fact that, far from spoiling a good walk in the woods, our middle-age status had brought us to an acceptance of our limitations and an understanding of what truly makes us tick at this age. Gone were the illusions that weighed us down in youth. Gone were the struggles of attaining success, and the prices we often paid. We were what we were this golden autumn day in Maine.

We skipped the back nine and had lunch. Ah, yes, middle age.

37

Amanda

Age does not protect you from love. But love, to some extent, protects you from age.

~ Jeanne Moreau

I don't know where John's relationship with Amanda will end up. They are the only ones who will have a say in that. I can offer no great words of wisdom to either foster their relationship or make them take a second look at it. So far removed from anything I ever experienced, the seventeen-year-old view of the world today is mystifying. Today's relationships between teens surely must also be. It is what it is, and, to John, it's good.

Amanda has found the key to John's heart. He tells her often, and without hesitation that he loves her. He is not bashful when he professes this and does not falter when stating it to her even in front of his parents. At first I thought John was all too cavalier with the way he casually threw around the word *love*. Seventeen-year-old boys, and for that matter girls, have feelings about what love must be, but it's the wisdom of years that painstakingly bring it into perspective. It's the experience of falling in and out of love that renders more meaning to the word.

But still, we all had our first loves. We all had that special person who even today we think back on fondly when present-day relationships sometimes challenge us. We think of the simplicity of that first love. We think about how easy it was to maintain and build upon. We think about the silly little things that, in our youth, we did together to make each other happy. And we sometimes ponder, *What if?*

I could no more be critical of John for his choice of words than I could be of my reservations about him saying it. To John, Amanda is the sun, the moon, and the stars all rolled into one tiny blond-headed package. She is his support. She takes the brunt of his bad moods, the effects of the treatment, and his need for having his buddies around him. They have a bond between them that seems to grow each day.

As November moved to December, they were constantly together, even if an hour was all that was available before one of them had to do something. She'd go with John to the treatment sessions adding to the support system that carried us along. They smiled and giggled at silly jokes and watched endless hours of television as John lay prostrate dealing with the fatigue. They bickered some; at times reminding me of classic sitcoms where the husband and wife are at odds during the program but always end in each other's arms by the end of the show.

Amanda is an angel sent to constantly remind John that there is comfort in someone other than his parents' arms. She is the rock he relies on for constancy. She allows John the normalcy of teenage life at a time when there is nothing normal in his life.

There is something naïve and innocent about John and Amanda's approach to life. Their simplistic view of the world comes from never having faced a mortgage, a crappy job, or a crying child in the middle of the night. These experiences and more will face them later and test them both. For now, I simply marvel at the ease of it, the things that make them happy, and, yes, the love they share.

38

Toy Soldiers

The desire to take medicine is perhaps the greatest feature which distinguishes man from animals.

~ Sir William Osler

Before John's illness, we decided to remodel our kitchen. In one corner, we created an area where I could do prep work for Nancy as she cooked. John's vast array of drugs takes up that space now. The bottles stand like tin soldiers on the pitch-black granite top ready to do battle. They are all specialists.

While void of fruits and vegetables and not used for its original intention, the counter serves a new purpose now. The counter is the pharmacy of life. I don't believe we will ever look at that counter the same way again. We wish for a day when the soldiers melt away and their battle is done.

For nausea:
    Granisetron (Kytril)
    Lorazepam (Ativan)
    Ondansetron (Zofran)
    Emend (to be given after Aloxi, administered by IV)
    Dronabinol (Marinol)
Cancer fighting steroid:
    Prednisone (very bad stuff)
Bacteria:
    Sulfamethoxazole (Bactrim)

For bowels:
Senna – C Plus
Stool softeners
Miralax
For pain:
Oxycodine
Oxycontine

Injected at various weeks in the chemo process, John received:
Nitrogen mustard
Vincristine
Bleomycin
Etopside
Adriamycin
Vinblastine

39

Media Hound

I wish people who have trouble communicating would just shut up.

~ Tom Lehrer

From a very early age, John had a presence. This was apparent on several occasions, but very much so when the cameras of the media were about. When I think back on two occasions when the spotlight shone upon him, I recall that he didn't flinch—he was a natural, and filled us with immense pride when we watched him.

I don't recall the grade, but it had to be the first or second grade when John did his first on-camera performance. It was Thanksgiving, and the media was out and about at the schools drumming up cute Thanksgiving stories from the children. They stopped at Hall Elementary School, which John attended, and interviewed the kids. When they settled on John, they asked him about what happens at his house on Thanksgiving. The interviewer went on to inquire if John enjoyed turkey.

"Yup, I like turkey," he responded.

"What do you do to make it taste good?" the reporter inquired.

"My mom puts grease on it," was his rather loud response.

Mom and Dad laughed so hard we almost peed our pants. The serious gourmet cook sitting beside me had chosen a moment of inquiry (when John had asked why she was rubbing butter on the outside of the turkey) to act silly around her impressionable son. Silly met silly as John took this as gospel and proceeded to tell the whole world his mother slathered something akin to breakfast renderings upon the sacred bird. With six innocent words we had learned our lesson.

Our second brush with immortality produced through the media was when John, at age twelve, gave a speech at City Hall. Earlier that month, a group of racists had left leaflets around the adjoining neighborhoods in response to Hall School and its incredibly expanded immigrant population. For whatever reason, these ignorant souls felt threatened by the diversity encompassing their neighborhoods. The students and staff fought back.

Chosen by his classmates to give a speech, John laid it on the line as he saw it. All the dignitaries were present when he spoke. There were cameras everywhere at the event. We kept a copy of his speech, and take pride to this day that he spoke from his heart:

"Some kids are skinny are some kids are not so skinny.

Some kids are short and some kids are tall.

Some kids are nice and some nicer.

Different languages, different color skin, it doesn't matter.

You know what? Different is just different.

We all belong at Hall School."

40

Are you ready For a Whole day, Dad?

The only thing that makes life possible is permanent, intolerable uncertainty; not knowing what comes next.

~ Ursula K. LeGuin

Nancy put the "Big Boy" tumor into perspective for me when she converted the metric measurements. Metrics to me were always a mystery as they are to most Americans of my generation. The tumor measured six inches long by three inches wide by four inches in depth. You can imagine this as slightly larger than a small sub roll.

On December 11, John was scheduled for a CT scan, a pulmonary test, and, of all things, a dental appointment. Nancy's time-off benefits had run out for the year. I would accompany John on these long-awaited appointments that would speak to how much progress the treatments had actually accomplished so far. My sincere wish to be on another planet that day never came true. I was stuck.

John knew what the day would involve, and knew that I had the duty as he announced the evening before, "Are you ready for a whole day, Dad?"

John was waiting to know, as we all were, if the whole business was doing any good at all. His knowledge of what was going on around him had swelled as the treatment process moved forward. You couldn't pull the wool over his eyes because he listened and took it all in. John decidedly knew the score on all counts. He was seventeen, and, yes, seventeen-year-old kids do lose perspective at times. He never did. He knew the entire process and understood the ramifications of success or failings in the treatment. He was ready and geared for whatever the outcome defined.

As we headed to the Maine Medical Radiology Center in Scarborough, the roads began icing over thanks to a persistent freezing rain. Adding to my anxious mode this morning, we now had to plod along behind cautious drivers on the Interstate. In the seat next to me, John sat in a stone-quiet mood. It had been barely two months since our nightmare had begun, and here we were heading off to get our first progress report.

Sitting in the waiting room with a geriatric crowd all waiting for X-rays, CT scans, MRIs, and PET scans, it dawned on me that John didn't fit in here. He was young, and they were all old. What the hell had brought us here? Childhood cancer had led us here, of course. The two words together sounded revolting. It was as if they didn't belong. Yet here we were with the old people waiting for our turn with the machine that would peer into John and expose what was going on.

The nurse quickly came for John, and off he went, leaving me with my newspaper, trying as I might to forget what secrets the CT scan could reveal. It wasn't long afterward that the nurse came and asked me to be with John as she had me sign some authorization forms. There he sat in his wool hat, a hospital johnnie, and a flimsy bathrobe looking for all the world as if someone had just squeezed all the life out of him. He was nauseous from the medicine he'd had to drink for the CT scan, and complained about being sweaty. The nurse handed him a vomit bag, and John left quietly for the bathroom as I signed the forms.

John's doctor ordered enhanced views of his CT scan. Whether John felt rotten or not, an IV was necessary to provide the substance required for the enhancement. If he felt terrible, he soon felt worse as the nurse missed the first vein entirely on his right arm and had to move to the left. I watched as he grimaced through the second arm as she lifted the needle time and again after it was securely in.

"What about the medi-port?" I asked.

"Oh, he has one?" she replied.

Obviously a rookie. We both hoped not to see her in the near future.

As I retreated to the room full of old people, I felt like complaining about the nurse, but I didn't. I simply sank into the industrially hard waiting room chair and waited. How much more of this can this poor kid take? His entire world seemed turned upside down. Once a week they shot him up with poison, scanned him with enough X-rays to make a horse sterile, and now they had stuck him in the wrong place. He'd suffered the embarrassment of his mother asking him for a semen sample, to be frozen in the event he became sterile. He'd lost his hair, he shuffled, missed too much school, his body was in pain, and rarely did a day go by when the nausea didn't remind him of the chemo. Gee, enough already, folks! Can't we take a break or something?

After sharing a very quick lunch, we were off to the Maine Medical Center for more tests. These breathing tests, as explained to me, would determine if the chemo had had any effect on his lungs. I didn't ask what the effects might be. How much worse could they be than cancer?

As John settled in for the test, he looked completely done in. He complained, as we walked from the parking garage, that his legs hurt, and he got testy with me for not finding the correct elevator as quickly as he thought I should have. The test was tedious and required John to give deep breaths into a tube. The constant cold he'd had for several weeks made it difficult. He got dizzy a couple of times, and the doctor let him rest. Thankfully, it was over soon, and we were on our way.

There was nothing else to do now except let him hit the couch and rest. We'd wait for the results of the CT scan that Dr. Rossi promised she would report to us later that day. Our father/son outing of this day would end in no good news or bad. There was nothing left to do but wait again.

As we drove home from the hospital, I reminded John that Mom would be home in time to get him to his dental appointment. He looked at me with a sneer and growled out, "You have to be kidding me, right?"

41

Small Victories

A mind troubled by doubt cannot focus on the course to victory.
~ Arthur Golden

The doctors hoped to see, in the CT scan, disappearance of the tumors as a result of the chemo. If this could be achieved, it was possible that the chemo could be stopped. The radiation therapy, which was scheduled for after the chemo, also might be cancelled.

More anxiety at the end of the day soon followed, mirroring the anxiety we had experienced at the start of our day. We waited for the phone call that would give us the news the same way we had waited through all the other fearful processes. We didn't want to think about what bad news we might receive; we couldn't talk to each other about it. We all went about our business the best we could until Nancy finally gave in and called the doctor's office. More disappointment followed. They would have to call her back. Again we waited.

We needed some good news, something to brighten everyone's spirits, something to help put us back on track. There had to be a light at the end of the tunnel. What about the odds, what about all the success stories? Surely we'd get some good news this time; surely we had all earned it.

When the call finally came, I listened intently from the next room. Nancy didn't say much, just an occasion "okay." It was over all too soon. The "wet" reading of the CT scan showed the chemo was shrinking the tumors. That was all the information they gave us from the results of what they call a "wet reading" of the CT scan. A discussion of the full results remained for the following week at John's next chemo session.

Now what? Was this a small victory or a major disappointment? Were we on the road to recovery, or was this a setback? I tried in vain to understand more about the phone conversation, but Nancy insisted I received all the information she had. We talked a bit more, and both of us decided to view this as a small victory. They hadn't disappeared, but, still, they had shrunk. The rest of the chemo and the radiation would take care of the remaining we insisted to each other.

Nancy put a positive spin on the results and informed John and Amanda. A few minutes later, as he shuffled past my door to the bathroom, I inquired of him, "Hey, good news isn't it, John?"

"Yeah, not bad" he replied.

That was a start. It was better than nothing. Our real hope now lay in the notion that John believed he was getting better, and all the work had not been a wasted effort. Showing progress we believed was paramount to his well-being. John's mind had to stay in "fix-it mode" to carry him through the rest of the treatments. He would need the same focus he had shown thus far.

42

Traditions

Traditions are the guideposts driven deep in our subconscious minds.
The most powerful ones are those we can't even describe, aren't even aware of.

~ Ellen Goodman

As remarkable as it may seem, there are still people in this fast-paced, high-tech, everyone-for-themself crazy world who still favor tradition over nonconformity. I'm one of them. I very much enjoy opening a car door for a women or sliding in a chair. I don't think it sexist, and, frankly, if she wants to do it for me, I'm okay with that too. It's simply a polite custom advanced over hundreds of years. I enjoy keeping and advancing traditions such as that.

The Deering High School / Portland High School turkey day game is a tradition. Over decades, it's served as a venue where long-lost alumni gather to celebrate their pasts and rekindling old friendships. I'm afraid that today, though, if the event were lost to budget cuts, there would at first be some grumbling, and then nothing. Many people don't favor tradition, especially if there's a price attached or it's something no one else is doing.

"Oh, how quaint, you have lobster stew each Christmas eve? How marvelous for you, darling."

When John was in kindergarten, Nancy and I decided to donate a sixty-five-foot Blue Spruce tree that had completely taken over a quarter of our front yard. The city accepted the tree, and, with much fanfare, it arrived in downtown Portland. A newspaper story soon followed. We were very proud that our family had played a part in the enjoyment of people that Christmas season by helping to keep a tradition alive in Portland.

From that day forward, John and I had our own Christmas tree tradition. Every year, we've shopped for our family's Christmas tree together. We head out on a Saturday morning a couple weeks before Christmas looking for "Nancy's tree." It can't be just any tree. It must be short (six foot is preferable) and stout. Bring a tall, skinny tree into the house and watch out. As John and I perfected our shopping technique, we came to find ourselves experts on the sizing up of a Christmas tree. We'd usually find our prize in a matter of minutes. Never did an unacceptable Christmas tree cross our threshold.

This year would be no different. With John looking like the ghost of Christmas past, and the temperature hovering around fifteen degrees (another tradition), we made our way to find the tree—with John driving. Our tree vendor's yard resembled a war zone, with the trees frozen in one large heap of needles and ice. We walked about for approximately forty-eight seconds and, once again, found the perfect tree—completely covered with ice from the storm the day before. I dragged it from its perch to the open yard and attempted to pay the person there, but I was told we'd have to go inside because they still had no power in the yard. As we waited in line, John asked for my gloves and said he was going to go load the tree.

"It's pretty heavy, John," was my response.

I was met with the familiar, "Whatever."

When I rejoined John, he had loaded the tree safely in the back of the pickup, but he remarked, "Wow, that was really bad, Dad."

"What, John?"

"Loading that damn tree took it all out of me."

From the time he was just a little kid, we had done this together. It was our tradition: father and son taking the time to enjoy each other in an all-too-brief moment for today's teenager. Today was special. In spite of his pain, his fatigue, and the cold air that tore through him, he mindfully kept the tradition going. He could have just stayed in bed and let me do it myself. I certainly would have understood. He didn't do that. He accepted our tradition because, to him, it was important, as important as anything else he was dealing with.

43

Public Servant

Hard work spotlights the character of people: some turn up their sleeves, some turn up their noses, and some don't turn up at all.

~ Sam Ewing

Nancy had gone to great lengths the past summer to ensure that John had employment. Working as she did at the courthouse, she had managed to wrangle him a summer job with the maintenance staff. His primary job would be to help on a special project: breaking up old concrete sidewalks and replacing them. The thought of his skinny little body doing hard manual labor for an extended period of time had me saying to myself with a chuckle, "Now he'll know exactly what's in store for him if he doesn't go to college."

Out of the gate, things started poorly. John suddenly came down with bronchitis the week he was supposed to start. He made it through one and half days, and they sent him home. The suddenness of this raised flags with both Nancy and me. It would not be the first time dear Johnny would play the "fake" card to avoid doing something. We badgered him that Sunday to get his act in gear and be at work on Monday. Of course, little did we know that this same bronchitis would return later and start us in motion. Had they missed some swollen lymph nodes when he went in for an antibiotic? Was his cancer already growing? In all likelihood, it was. No one will ever know for sure.

With Ryan, a newly minted Bates College graduate firmly ensconced as John's supervisor, and a good paying job in hand, we had visions of John accepting the responsible position as perhaps a new look at the world outside his friends, and a means by which he could fully accept the concept of, "a fair day's work for a fair day's pay." We learned quickly that county maintenance jobs, while they did pay well, were not that filled with either responsibility or a robust work ethic. John's first day of work involved a barbeque at the county jail and a quest for steel-toed boots. When we asked how much work he'd done, he looked at us quizzically and said, "Work?"

John soon flourished as just another one of the "crew" in this blue-collar environment. Much to John's dismay, plenty of work stood in front of him. The work was hard, and he'd settle in at home afterward with the aches and pains of muscles used too sparingly in the past. But always he'd gather enough energy to hang out with his buds in the evening. The notion of too much work and too little play did not enter John's mind. With pocket money now in plentiful supply, and not having to twenty-dollar his parents to death, John envisioned a consumer summer—indeed, a fun time.

We forced him to put money away, even managing it for him when it became evident that he'd found it a simple feat to blow through a hundred dollars in a weekend or less. He fought the notion saying it was his money, and that he had worked hard for it. True, but, with direct deposit, we held all the cards.

Although the focus remained on sidewalk reconstruction, John occasionally received other assignments. One of these involved motoring to Massachusetts with a co-worker to pick up two sheriff's patrol cars. These were not just any cars. Decked-out-ready-to-go patrol cars is what they were. It boggles the mind to understand why any sane human being would heap this much responsibility on a seventeen-year-old with a license less than six months old in his pocket. But they did. Nancy asked if he and his buddy had put the lights on.

"Only in the rest area," was his reply.

I asked in kind, "So, how fast, John?"

"One hundred, I guess."

"Great, John. What are you, nuts?"

"What?"

"Do you know how much trouble you could be in?"

This was just not sinking in, and I couldn't help but laugh at the lunacy of it all. Good idea? I think not. I could read the headlines now. What were these people thinking?

When he got back to the city, he still couldn't leave well enough alone. Passing a local police car, John waited for the officer to wave first because he thought, in the hierarchy of police people, a deputy sheriff was more important than a local policemen. He did, however, at least have the good sense to finally wave back.

With the great police car caper ending, life went back to normal for the hardworking summer crew. Lunch was the highlight of the day. It was here that John got to listen to the lives of just plain working people. He stayed in the background at first, but with time soon became a lunchroom favorite. They played paper football, and John won the title. John bet his mates they couldn't eat seven Saltine crackers in a minute, and soon the challenge went through the courthouse. No one ever did, but John got the closest with six.

One luncheon brought John firmly into the fold when a worker known for his bellicose ways insisted that, if a fat person and a skinny person fell off a Ferris wheel together, the fat person would land first. John quickly stood on a chair and dropped two bottles of soda—one empty and one full. They both landed together. With his quirky little grin, he just said, "Wrong, it's physics."

The final remembrance John left with his co-workers was a vision of the county pickup truck after he'd jammed it into the exit of the parking garage. Ho-hum, just another day in the life of a county worker.

44

Couch Duty

Failure or success seems to have been allotted to men by their stars.
But they retain the power of wriggling, of fighting with their star
or against it, and in the whole universe the only really interesting
movement is this wriggle.

~ E. M. Forster

John spent the better part of December on the living room couch.
With Amanda constantly by his side, they'd go through an endless
array of movies and television shows. They'd eat on the couch and only
move to go lie down in his room. Fatigue was taking a toll on him both
physically and mentally. He didn't speak often, and, when he did, it
was in hushed tones. A shower was the most physically taxing exercise
he could manage. He would rarely now make more than two classes a
day at school if he managed to go at all.

Even with the good news we had gotten this week from his radiologist
regarding the shrinking tumors, he just showed no enthusiasm or
spirit. The medicine was beating him up pretty badly, but, with the last
treatment of the "mustard" having been given, we thought he'd perk up
a bit and know that he was in the home stretch. He just didn't. He was
always in pain. The medicines helped in so far as they took the edge off,
but pain was a constant at this point. He moved like an old man and
rarely did anything that required him to exert himself. A cold he'd had
for weeks made him feel all that much worse, and the doctors wouldn't
allow us to give him anything for it because they feared it might affect

the chemo. For the first time in the ordeal, I saw him losing his edge and wondered if he had chosen to stop fighting.

The first big snowstorm of the year dumped sixteen miserable inches of snow on us a week before Christmas. During the past winter, John had taken over the snow blower detail for me. Trying to inject some humor, I reminded him that the spring storms would be all his again. Having tried to start the beast for the past two days with no success, I held my breath as I finally, gently, coxed the thing to life. If it didn't start, I had no doubt they'd find the three of us in the spring clutching a jar of olives—the last food in the house—in a death grip.

As I cleared the driveway using muscles I hadn't used in a very long time, I thought of John languishing on the couch and I wondered what he was thinking about my doing his chore. It's hard to imagine being that young, and so physically undone by something not of his choice.

Christmas was creeping up on us fast. John's stepbrother Aaron would be arriving from New Mexico two days after Christmas with his girlfriend Elizabeth. Over the years, Aaron had become closer with John—a good big brother—and John looked up to him. Aaron always made a point to include John, regardless of the age difference. While John didn't show much emotion about the visit, we could tell he wanted his brother there. He'd spent so much time with Amanda that having another guy around would certainly be good medicine. I think he instinctively knew it too.

We'd talked to Aaron repeatedly over the past few weeks bringing him up to date on John's condition and letting him know what to expect. Aaron is a good kid. He's the type of kid who has to do everything himself without outside help. His latest adventure proved to be just the type of thing he loved to do. Aaron loves to cook and is good at it. He'd taken a job with a catering company in New Mexico that worked on movie sets feeding the cast and crew. On each movie he'd meet a new star, and, with much fanfare, he'd tell us all about his encounters. He was excited about coming for Christmas and knew what to expect. We had no doubt he would brighten all our lives.

With the pain and fatigue, also came the anger and hostility. It wasn't a constant. It would jump out at you at any given moment with such emotion you never knew what to expect next. It wasn't John. The frustration of the situation and the emotions he carried inside through the ordeal left him with no one to vent against except Amanda and his parents. As the chemo worked its magic, it also worked its best to make John into a different person at times. With each outburst, followed later by an apology, the mood swings became second nature to all of us.

The ups became fewer while the downs seemed to heap more and more weight on his skinny shoulders. We'd followed the Giants all that fall watching them successfully make the playoffs. John's excitement was tempered when two back-to-back evening games went unwatched as he begrudgingly made his way off to bed at a time when, in the past, he'd just be leaving for an evening of revelry with his friends. Sleep was his ally, one of many allies he could count on as a constant in his battle.

45

A Christmas Gift

And the Grinch, with his Grinch-feet ice cold in the snow, stood puzzling and puzzling, how could it be so? It came without ribbons. It came without tags. It came without packages, boxes or bags. And he puzzled and puzzled 'till his puzzler was sore. Then the Grinch thought of something he hadn't before. What if Christmas, he thought, doesn't come from a store. What if Christmas, perhaps, means a little bit more.

~ Dr. Seuss

December 24, 2008, would see John shuffle off for his tenth chemo treatment since October. The treatment would be a mild medicine, and we were thankful and hopeful it would not wreak havoc with him on Christmas Eve and the following day. The plan called for us to travel to my sister's for Christmas day if John was up to it. The entire family of aunts, uncles, nieces, nephews, grandchildren, and parents would descend on her home to celebrate.

Nancy had completed the gift buying with a few final items that morning. Truth be told, we both just wanted the holiday to come and go so we could settle back into the routine of tending to John. The special part of this Christmas would be the knowledge that John's fight was succeeding, the chemo was doing its job, and that we were grateful for the huge support system of people who continued to help make our job, if not easier, then somewhat less painful.

Still, there were things that needed to be done; chief among them was cleaning the bathroom, the one chore in the house that neither

Nancy nor I wanted to do. I took it upon myself to accomplish the task when the room seemed to have gone too long without a thorough hosing. With all the necessary cleaning supplies, I dove into it as Nancy and John left for his treatment. As do most men, I do a far better job of messing up a bathroom than I do at cleaning one. But for some reason that day, I'd resolved to clean the thing as if it contained some horrible plague rather than a bit of soap scum and a few strands of hair. The whole thing made me mad all of a sudden. For two months, we'd had little time to devote to anything but John. The house had suffered, work had taken a backseat, take-out food had become the norm, and emotions were all over the board. Clean? I'll show you clean!

As I successfully finished my task, the group returned from the cancer center.

"How'd you do, John?" I greeted him.

"Okay," he answered—his usual reply.

"How are you feeling?" I said trying to coax more out of him.

"All right, I guess."

Well, so much for trying to get information or show some concern. It didn't matter; I'd query Nancy after she took her coat off and got settled in. Trouble was, she was ready to head off someplace again.

"So, how did it go?" I asked the same question I'd asked for weeks.

"There's no activity."

"What do you mean, there's no activity? What the hell does that mean?"

"Just what I said, there's no activity," she responded. "It's gone. The tumors don't show up on the PET anymore."

"Gone? You mean completely? What did Dr. Rossi say?"

"She gave me a high five, hugged me, and said Merry Christmas!"

And with that, Nancy gave me a high five, hugged me, said Merry Christmas, and rushed out the door as John and Amanda headed upstairs.

Wait a minute. I'm standing here all alone after getting the news we had been waiting for since this whole ordeal started. What the hell am I doing here alone? Doesn't anyone want to celebrate? Doesn't anyone want to join me as I run up and down Stevens Avenue screaming at the top of my lungs, "Thank you, Lord!"?

I'd asked John how it had gone, and he'd responded with "okay." For crying out loud, what the hell does "okay" mean nowadays? I'd hate to see what it would take to make him respond with something like "marvelous." And Nancy—she either didn't fully understand what she'd just said to me, or she was in shock.

"Come back here, all of you! Let's sit down and think for a minute what this all means. Can't we at least hug and cry for a few minutes?"

As I sat down by the Christmas tree, next to a warming fire, I contemplated the madness of the past two months and what we still had left to accomplish. In the short time of the journey's duration, from the turning of the leaves of autumn to the first snows of winter, we had encountered feelings of such magnitude they would change all of our lives forever. We had experienced so much love and kindness from family, friends, and co-workers that, at times, it overwhelmed us. Simple, spontaneous acts brightened our day when the darkness of the moment seemed ready to swallow us all. All of the "what ifs" seemed to disappear now with the clarity and certainty of the day's news and the comfort of knowing we were winning the fight.

As I sipped a glass of wine alone, warm in my world by the fire, I felt good. It was Christmas Eve; God had answered the prayers.

Epilouge

When you come to the end of all the light you know, and it's time to step into the darkness of the unknown, faith is knowing that one of two things shall happen: Either you will be given something solid to stand on or you will be taught to fly.

~ Edward Teller

There were no balloons, and no marching bands. The ordeal seemed to stop as quickly as it had started with the three of us shaking our heads and saying to each other, "What the hell just happened?"

It's March 2, 2009. We've moved into a new year. Another foot of snow fell today, adding to the winter's endless total. This "winter of our discontent" seems to drag on at a pace that would test anyone's mettle, and add to the burden we have carried since the first flakes fell. However, things are plainly different. Today, as he did after the past couple of storms, John shoveled the front walk and raked the back roof.

The journey that has encompassed all of us since Christmas has been a time of success and encouragement. There is virtually no bad news to report. John is recovering in fine fashion. While the radiation treatments left him weak and fatigued, he has begun to function as a teenager again. He saw the "light at the end of the tunnel" and responded with the enthusiasm of youth. While his appetite is still shot, and he can't go any length of time without resting, his smile is back, his hair is growing, his eyebrows have reappeared, and he is out and about with his "buds" as if the whole thing was nothing more than a slight interruption in his life. His sense of humor, something Nancy and I always enjoyed, came back with the same, familiar quirkiness.

Cancer patients aren't told, but instinctively know, that, when they are scheduled to have their medi-port removed, the doctors feel that they have reached the point when they have beaten back the disease, when they believe that no further injections of any kind are needed. For Nancy and me, it was the point when our breathing became normal again, and talks about college started to replace talks about the next treatment. For John, it was a time when blood tests, chemo, and all the poking and prodding would be replaced with the normalcy of attending school on a regular basis and returning to a simple and understandable world.

How did all this happen? What carried us through this? Why, in the short time frame from October to March had we come from an incredible diagnosis, to the astounding place we are today? It's maddening to assume that someone or something played a bigger part in all this. Talks about guardian angels, faith, support from everyone, confidence in modern medicine, and just plain luck, occurred over and over again throughout the process. Did one carry the day? It's not for me or anyone else to say. It is what it is. Or is it? Do miracles have a place in our lives? Do we rely on other powers that, as mortals, we fail to comprehend? Who can say? Do things such as this happen as a test, or are they just part of a universe of happenings that blend to form the human spirit?

We're all exhausted. The energy required and expended has been enormous. It drained us all to the extent that everything else was put on hold. We found that together, supporting each other, we could achieve the true spirit of family. John matured through the ordeal. And Nancy expanded on her "Super Mom" persona. For me, it was the notion that Dad had to be Dad. How could I change in the midst of such events? Humor, constant focus on the facts as they came to light, and, much to my chagrin, straightforward talk with no bullshit helped me handle a situation that, at times, was totally out of my control. At times, John cringed at the things I had to say. Other times, I'd manage a wry smile from him at a time when the pain was his only focus. I tried my best to understand and to show John that Dad was there. Never through the whole process did I feel as if John would cave in. He was so courageous from beginning to end that I never felt the need to sugarcoat anything.

He would have seen right through anything of this nature, and the process would have slowed to a crawl.

John has drifted in and out of school the past few months, always maintaining his honor-roll status. This was by no means an easy feat, as he could have just dumped it all and no one would have cared in the least. His achievements say a lot about his character and what he thinks is important. Doing homework at a time when he just wanted to go to bed and forget about the events of the day brought out his toughness and resilience. The second semester is equally off to a good start, although he did dump advanced-placement history, claiming he had to have fewer subjects to really concentrate on them and do well. Under mild objection, we caved in and allowed him to make his own decision.

John will see his eighteenth birthday in May. This unofficial start of manhood was once something we didn't talk about lest our hopes were shattered. Odd as it may seem, when he turns eighteen, we are no longer in charge of his health. We can't sign forms, dictate treatment, or give clearances. His age dictates that he must do that himself. So what's in a number? Is he ready to take on the responsibility of making decisions for himself? I think he is.

John's friends, especially Amanda, stuck with him through the ordeal. I would often come home to find a bedroom full of his mates wailing over some video game. The camaraderie associated with youth withstood the insidious disease and still flourishes. I don't know what his friends thought to see him bald and so sick. I'd like to think they all took stock and recalled the saying, "There but for the grace God go I." I'd like to think they all became better human beings from witnessing such an event. I'd like to think they will better understand if a loved one is ever given a similar diagnosis. I'd like to think their experience with John will help them if the time ever comes when they have to deal with it again. I know it will.

Writing this narrative was painful, while, at the same time, exhilarating. Never did I think I could open myself to pen and paper and expose my feelings to friends, family, and colleagues. As witnessed by what you have just read, I'm not a writer. There is no technical skill I profess to have. The notion that I could ever fashion anything beyond business writing left me at times wanting to stop for fear of how this work would be accepted. But, it was too important to put aside. It doesn't matter if the sentence structure is wrong. It doesn't matter if my thoughts wander to the point where even I didn't understand what I was trying to say at times. I had to write this for John. He has to know how we felt, how we dealt with the pain, and how we desperately wanted an end to our son's struggle.

There are still challenges that lie ahead. John will be tested on a regular basis for many years, if not for a lifetime. Could he relapse? No one knows. What we do know is that we all feel confident we did the best possible with something that was thrown into our lives at a time when no one even gave a thought to the possibility that something like it could happen. The three of us used whatever we had to make sure this bad dream would leave our lives as quickly as it entered.

I'm so proud. I'm proud of Nancy, proud of our friends, family, and everyone else who shared this journey with us. You all know who you are and what you contributed. You guided us, consoled us, cried with us, and always made us feel that we weren't alone. You never held back.

As we move into John's senior year, and graduation fever takes hold, we can only marvel at the events that have led us to this day. I will undoubtedly embarrass myself when I stand and cheer when John's name is announced. To me, the achievement will be something that speaks for itself, something beyond words, and something worth screaming at the top of my lungs for. So when that day comes, John, don't be embarrassed by your dad and his antics.

Laugh with Mommy and I, and make it your purpose in life to be a better person because of this journey back. Never ever change the person you are. Find love and grow old with your mate. Always remember this brief moment in your life as a journey back to new beginnings, and a time you faced with the courage and wisdom of someone beyond your years.

On Mother's Day, May 10, 2009, Nancy received her customary letter from John. He knows that every year this is all she wants from him. This is what John wrote:

Another year has gone by since I've written you your Mother's Day letter, and what a year it's been. Let me say that again, what a year it's been! There were times when I was more scared than I've ever been, but with you around, Mom, I knew nothing could hurt me. Through every terrible chemo moment you were there, along with the surgeries and check-ups. I am so grateful to have a mother who is always thinking of me before herself. I really can't put into words how lucky I feel that I have such a wonderful, loving mummy.

Even when Amanda was gone and it was late at night, you slept with an ear and eye open for any distress from your sick son. There is simply no way I could have endured through such misery without you by my side, Mom. I feel as though my having cancer brought our family closer together inside the house. All those tough moments helped us realize the joy we find in one another. I think of it as a blessing, really, because it helped me appreciate life and family more than I thought possible. Mom, I love you so much and could not have made it through that horrible stuff without you by my side. Thank you so much for birthing me and caring for me daily. Happy Mother's Day.

Johnny

List Of Quoted Authors

Penelope Leach (1937–) British child development specialist

Alexandre Dumas (1802–1870) Author

Hervey Allen (1889–1949) Novelist, poet, and biographer

Dave Barry (1947–) US humorist and columnist

Al McGuire (1928–2001) Basketball coach and TV commentator

Carl Sandburg (1878–1967) Poet

Erma Bombeck (1927–1996) Author and columnist

E.V. Lucas (1868–1938) Author and critic

Charles Osgood (1933–) Radio and television commentator

King Edward VIII (1894–1972) King of England

Denis Diderot (1713–1784) Encyclopedic

Edna St. Vincent Millay (1892–1950) Poet and author

Ralph Waldo Emerson (1803–1882) Poet and author

Jeff Foxworthy (1958–) Actor and comedian

Thomas Szasz (1920–) Psychiatrist

Jacqueline Kennedy Onassis (1929–1994) First Lady of the United States

Heather Armstrong (1975–) Blogger

Martha Washington (1732–1802) First Lady of the United States

Heywood Broun (1888–1939) Sports reporter, commentator

Anne Rice (1941–) Author

Mark Twain (1835–1910) Author

Tom Stoppard (1937–) Playwright

Scott Adams (1957–) Cartoonist

Erica Jong (1942–) Author

Charles Haddon Spurgeon (1834–1892) English Baptist preacher

Cyril Connolly (1903–1974) English critic and editor

Helen Keller (1880–1968) Author, activist, and lecturer

John Wayne (1907–1979) Actor

Dorothy Parker (1893–1967) Author, humorist, and poet

John Powell (1925–) Educator and author

Sam Levenson (1911–1980) Humorist and writer

Epes Sargent (1813–1881) Poet

Louis D. Brandeis (1856–1941 Justice, U.S. Supreme Court

Scott Westerfeld (1953–) Author

Jim Morrison (1943–1971) Poet and singer

Albert Einstein (1879–1955) Physicist

Jeanne Moreau (1928–) Actress

Sir William Osler (1849–1919) Physician

Tom Lehrer (1928–) Mathematician, composer, and satirist

Ursula K. LeGuin (1929–) Author and poet

Arthur Golden (1957–) Journalist and writer

Ellen Goodman (1941–) Columnist

Sam Ewing (1949–) Professional baseball player

E. M. Forster (1879–1970) Novelist

Theodore Geisel (Dr. Seuss) (1904–1991) Writer and cartoonist

Edward Teller (1908–2003) Theoretical physicist

Meister Eckhart (1260–1328) Philosopher

www.ingramcontent.com/pod-product-compliance
Lightning Source LLC
Chambersburg PA
CBHW061305280526
45784CB00002B/903